PHYSICAL THERAPY RECRUITMENT BOOK

THE PHYSICAL THERAPY HIRING SOLUTION

HOW TO <u>RECRUIT</u>, <u>HIRE</u> AND <u>TRAIN</u>
WORLD-CLASS PEOPLE YOU CAN TRUST

PAUL GOUGH

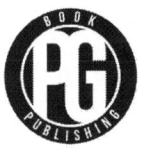

Paul Gough Publishing

Copyright © 2018 Paul Gough. All rights reserved.

This publication is licensed to the individual reader only. Duplication or distribution by any means, including email, disk, photocopy, and recording, to a person other than the original purchaser, is a violation of international copyright law.

Publisher: Paul Gough, 25 Raby Road, Hartlepool, UK, TS24 8AS

While they have made every effort to verify the information here, neither the author nor the publisher assumes any responsibility for errors in, omissions from or a different interpretation of the subject matter. This information may be subject to varying laws and practices in different areas, states, and countries. The reader assumes all responsibility for the use of the information.

The author and publisher shall in no event be held liable to any party for any damages arising directly or indirectly from any use of this material. Every effort has been made to accurately represent this product and its potential and there is no guarantee that you will earn any money using these techniques.

ISBN: 9781728900285

DEDICATION

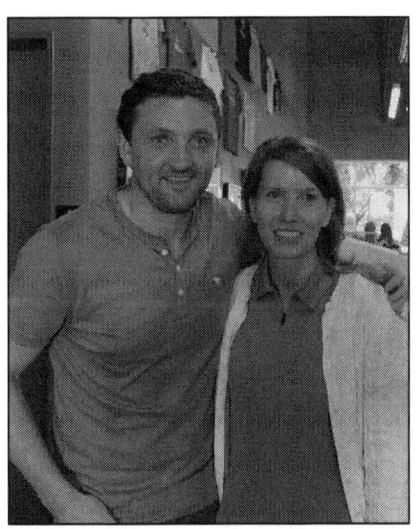 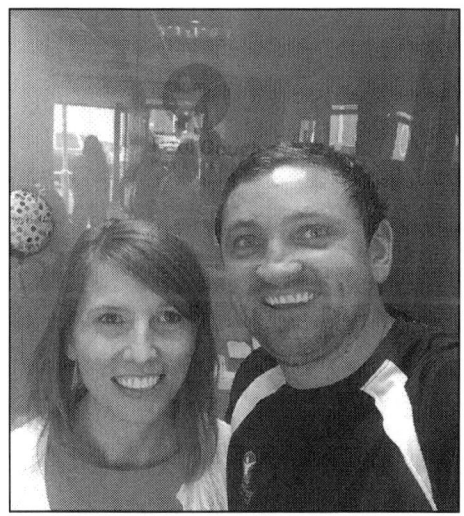

With Lois at her clinic in Phoenix, USA

With Lois at my clinic in Hartlepool, UK

This book is dedicated to the memory of Lois Wolff – top physical therapist and founder of AZ SportsCenter, Phoenix.

Lois was an amazingly kind and caring person who I had the pleasure to work with professionally and get to know personally.

Not long before her sudden death, Lois came all the way out to the UK from Phoenix to visit my clinic and it was my honor and privilege to spend time with her in my hometown of Hartlepool. A sudden illness in 2017 took her life way too early.

RIP Lois.

BEFORE YOU READ THE BOOK DO THIS FIRST...

Just to say thanks for reading this book **I would like to give you the Worksheets, Example Job Ads, Success Descriptions, and Top 10 Interview Questions PDF (plus "lost chapter" on how to fire!)** that are mentioned inside the book – absolutely FREE!

Go to:
www.paulgough.com/hiring-resource
to download it now.

Here's What You Will Receive:

- **My No.1 performing Job Ads** - just copy, tweak and paste into your next hiring campaign

- **The top 10 interview questions** – discover how to create the right questions to ask candidates, to determine if they're the right fit

- **Complete resources from the book** - including the success description templates and even more bonuses that I haven't mentioned here

It's All Here:
www.paulgough.com/hiring-resorce

YOU'LL NEED THIS AS YOU READ THE BOOK...

Go to: **www.paulgough.com/hiring-resource** now and download your FREE bonus Hiring Resource PDF – it contains many of the resources (and more) that I mention in the book...

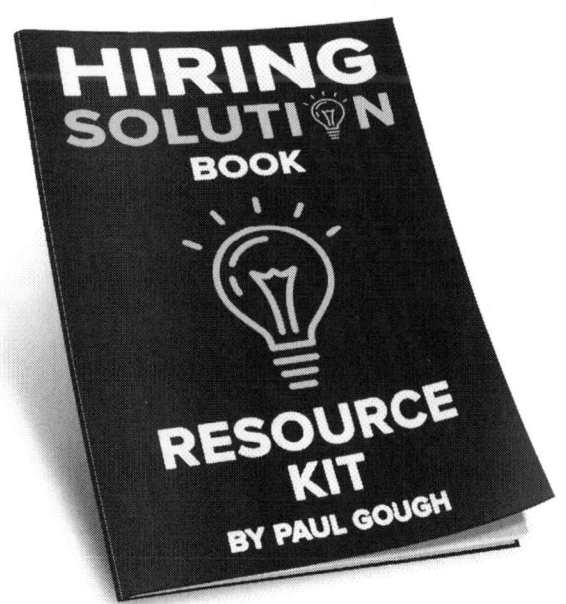

To get the best out of this book download the resource PDF now before you start reading:
www.paulgough.com/hiring-resoure

GET YOUR FREE WEALTH MARKETING GIFT FROM PAUL, NOW...

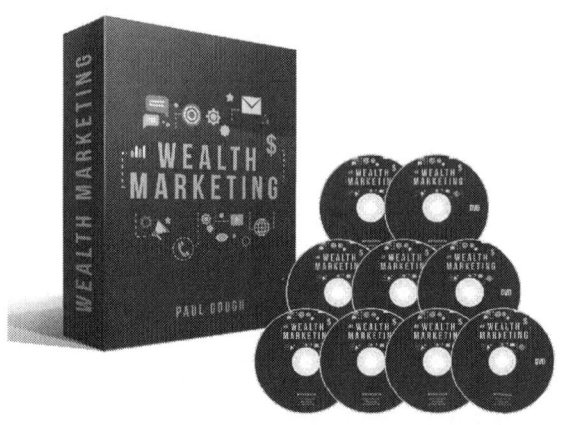

Go to: **www.paulgough.com/wealth-gift**
To get this instant access 9 DVD video program, NOW

Claim your $1,997.00 worth of cash patient generating, higher profit making, wealth marketing DVD program, absolutely FREE!

Including a FREE "Test-Drive" of Paul Gough's Cash Club Membership that sends to your clinic $10,000 worth of marketing ideas every 30 days.

**Claim your copy now, at
www.paulgough.com/wealth-gift**

CONTENTS

CHAPTER 1

Could Everything You've Ever Been Told

About Hiring Be Wrong? - 7

CHAPTER 2

The Biggest Hiring Mistake I Ever Made

(That Cost Me $100,000's...) - 25

CHAPTER 3

The Structure Of All World-class Companies - 45

CHAPTER 4

Who To Hire And When - 61

CHAPTER 5

Step 1/6: How To Create Your Hiring Plan - 81

CHAPTER 6

Step 2/6: How To Establish The Financial Metric

Of Success For A New Hire - 99

CHAPTER 7

Step 3/6: How To Create Your Success Description
(Outcomes, Tasks, Measure, Skills) - 107

CHAPTER 8

Step 4/6: How To Create Your Job Ad - 131

CHAPTER 9

Step 5/6: Where To Post Your Job Ad (11 Different Places) - 145

CHAPTER 10

Step 6/6: The Interview Process
(And What Questions To Ask) - 163

CHAPTER 11

Your Foolproof 7, 30 And 90 Day Onboarding Process – 195

CHAPTER 12

Case Study: How To Automate The Hiring Process - 219

CHAPTER 13

Your Opportunity To Work With Paul Beyond This Book - 235

INTRODUCTION

There's an argument that says if you employ the right people, then all of your business problems will be solved. And I agree.

Think about it: if you have a marketing problem, it can be solved by hiring a great marketer. If you have a sales and conversion issue, it can be solved by hiring a great sales person. If you have a cash flow issue, it can be solved by hiring the right financial controller. If your business is operating inefficiently, hiring a great operational manager can solve that.

In theory, you can, quite literally, hire your way out of problems.

But here's a key point: hiring to solve problems only works if you know what problem you've actually got. In truth, many business owners don't know that, and this is *the* problem they face each day.

I believe that your business success is defined by how good you are at solving the real problems at hand. Instead of blaming governments, insurance companies, the local economy, corporate hospitals – even POPTS – you will be more successful if you focus on solving the problem that all of those things expose.

What most clinic owners call problems are really symptoms; the root cause of the symptoms is often a failure to hire correctly; a failure to hire in order to solve the problem their business has.

For example, is the problem that you can't get enough leads? Or, is it that you don't have the right person doing the marketing for you? Did you employ your best friend's 21-year-old daughter to do your marketing just because she likes being on social media?

Is the problem that no one wants to pay out of pocket for your services? Or, is it that you hired a front desk person who is nice and polite, but has no clue how to handle objections to money?

Is the problem culture? Or is it that you employed a clinically gifted therapist to run your practice, yet one who is devoid of any ability to manage people, measure results, and call it tight in a way that others respect?

What's more, most clinic owners confuse "*how*" problems with "*who*" problems and end up sentencing themselves to a lifetime of perpetual struggle.

You might not know <u>how</u> to create the marketing system to bring in all of the new leads that you need. But guess what? There's someone out there <u>who</u> does. You might not know <u>how</u> to manage people. But guess what? There's someone out there <u>who</u> does. Employ the right person and free yourself up to lead your company if that is what you're better at.

THE TRADITIONAL METHODS FOR HIRING ARE FLAWED

I put it to you that your #1 obstacle in business growth is hiring. That's why I am glad you picked up this book when you did.

This is the second of a series of books that I'm writing for the global physical therapy business owner/private practice community. The first book was on *Marketing*, and it should not be lost on you that this second book is on *Hiring*. That's because most people who have read my first book about marketing, *"New Patient Accelerator Method"*, will by now have a new problem: acquiring staff to deal with a massive increase in the volume of phone calls and inquires that getting good at marketing causes.

(What a great problem to have!)

New Patient Accelerator exposed the traditional marketing methods for clinic owners as being flawed and out of date. It showed that statistically, chasing referrals from doctors is a complete waste of time – there's not enough go around. Besides, doing so keeps you trapped inside of a system with *decreasing* reimbursements and *increasing* expenses (more work, less profit).

And, relying upon word of mouth for your referrals sounds nice in theory, but is slow and unreliable in reality. You cannot grow or scale a business on slow and unpredictable.

Which brings us to this book...

<u>The traditional methods for hiring are also flawed and out of date.</u>

After years of "hiring for personality" and defaulting to experience, hiring *STILL* remains the no.1 headache for business owners.

The traditional methods of hiring will have you believe, that if you find someone with a nice personality who brings experience to the table, then all of your problems will be solved.

Having a great personality is important, but it doesn't come in handy when there's no money in the bank to meet payroll.

And as for experience, just because they have spent twenty-two years answering the phone for someone else, it doesn't automatically mean that they can handle the job in the way you need, or even that they're willing to learn how!

Successful hiring is, first and foremost, about solving a business problem; achieving an **outcome**.

To solve problems at scale, i.e. to grow, you need people to work together in tandem. This is often referred to as "culture". To achieve the culture that you want, you need people who share similar **values**. It has nothing whatsoever to do with personality.

I get the premise of the "hire for personality" idea, but it is fundamentally flawed. That's because personalities do not solve business problems – skills do. It is only when people with skills work together in tandem that you get problems solved and your business grows.

To know what **skills** you need, you first need to know what problems your business has; what are the **outcomes** that must be achieved? To achieve these outcomes, you need to know the **tasks** required of the outcome, and, to make sure the tasks are being done right, you need to **measure.**

These four steps make up what I call the *Hiring Success Triangle*, and they are just some of the things we will be covering in this book. The *Hiring Success Triangle* is an integral part of the *Outcomes Based Hiring System* that I created. It is a massive shift away from hiring for personality and experience – traditional methods doomed to fail – to hiring for **outcomes**, achieved by people with the right **skills,** and who have shared **values**.

Sounds a lot better already, doesn't it?

Be prepared… in the pages of this book I will be presenting to you a radically different approach to hiring; one that is different from anything you've ever tried before. It is the same approach that has allowed me to assemble a team of people I can trust to run my business in my absence. Since its conception, I've taught this approach to 100's of other clinic owners, and many have achieved the same freedom, security, and prosperity through applying it.

You'll learn that there's a big difference between employees "working hard" and actually achieving a specific outcome, such as, for example, improving your clinics arrival rate.

You'll stop thinking that just because someone has a good resume, or has experience, that they're right for your role. Likewise, you'll also learn how to spot people with no experience who *are* right for your role.

You'll learn how to identify your major outcomes for each role required – and hire people skilled enough to achieve them for you while being able to hold them accountable for it.

What's, you'll learn how to ask the right questions of candidates during an interview. This will take you closer to the people who share your values and are simultaneously able to perform as you need.

Ultimately, you're about to discover a system that will hand deliver the right employee; someone one who is able (and willing) to solve your problems while still being a pleasure to be around each day.

Enjoy the journey you're about to go on. I'll be taking you from confused, anxious, stressed, and worried about hiring, to enjoying the process knowing that the biggest problem in your business – hiring - is soon to be solved.

Let's begin the book…

1

COULD EVERYTHING YOU'VE EVER BEEN TOLD ABOUT HIRING BE WRONG?

I live by the belief that everything popular is **wrong**. As in, if everyone agrees that something is "the best way" then it most likely isn't. It is most likely the *easy* way, but that doesn't mean it is the most productive or most profitable.

And in the case of hiring, the popular belief is that that you "hire for personality" and "train for skill." It's as if the person who is happiest or smiles the most is automatically the right person for the job, regardless of whether or not they even have the skills required of the role.

I wonder just how many Major League Baseball players have been employed because of having a great personality?

The "hire for personality" thing sounds great on paper; it is a popularized way of thinking that allows business owners to short-cut needing to grasp the real needs of their businesses.

On the face of it, it is much quicker and easier to choose a candidate who smiles politely in an interview than it is to sit and think about what problems your business has actually got. It takes time to consider if the person smiling at you is able to solve your business problem and time is not always the friend of a business owner in a hiring situation. But just because something is quick and easy – that doesn't make it right.

Focusing solely on the person, and whether they have a great personality or not is flawed. How can I confidently say so? Because the "hire for personality" thing has been around for years and yet the biggest problem for most business owners is still finding and hiring the right people. There's a lot of happy, smiley candidates arriving for interviews these days and there are equally as many miserable business owners. I wonder what the link could be...

Hiring is every business owner's biggest headache, and yet it is the one part of the business that if you get right, makes running a business so much easier.

If you're like most clinic owners, I suspect there's rarely a day or week that goes by when you're not thinking, "if I just had better staff, then everything would be ok." Or, like so many do, blaming all of your current business struggles on the incompetency of the people you work with - the people you hired. The same people who you were certain at the time of hiring had the right personality that would have made them a success in your clinic.

If you've ever felt that way then you're not alone and I am so glad you picked up this book. I can tell you from experience that having the right people on your team makes your life so much easier. It also makes your business more successful. For some owners, getting the right people on board is the only thing standing in the way of more profit and more success.

But here's the thing: one of the worst things you can do is to daydream about finding better staff. Do not allow yourself to believe that better staff are growing on a tree somewhere and when you find it you can just go and pick them off. Or, even worse, allowing yourself to believe that you're so unlucky in life and business that you always miss out on the best staff – just because it is you!

People regularly look at my staff and assume that "I'm lucky" to have them. As if somehow, I am a magnet for attracting all of the best staff in any town that I set up a business. I can assure you that is not the case. The truth is that there's no such thing as a herd of world-class people all ready and willing to walk through your doors. There isn't some evil plot to keep the best ones from you, and there isn't a website where all of the world's best employees go to that you don't know about.

There is, however, a system for finding people and turning them into world-class performers that up until now, has not come your way. The reality of hiring world-class people is that it is as much about the system you use, as it is who you're looking for. If you want world-class people (the effect), then what you need is a world-class system of recruiting, hiring, and training that transforms them into a world-class member of staff (the cause).

That is what this book will give you.

WHO AM I AND HOW DID I LEARN THIS NEW SYSTEM?

My name is Paul Gough, and when I opened my first physical therapy clinic I thought I had it all figured out; I thought that my "superior" clinical skills would be enough to build a world-class business, one which makes a ton of profit. I soon learned that great clinical skills get you started, but they also get you stuck!

When I realized that I needed to learn how to *market* my practice, I went away and I did that. In fact, I did it so well that I found myself with a host of new problems that I hadn't bargained for as a trained physical therapist. And one of them was staff!

Specifically, getting the right staff in place to support the vision I had for my business. Getting the right people who could deliver the high-quality service *I* was already providing to my patients, soon become my biggest challenge.

As you will learn in this book, I got my first hire right – but it was more by luck than by design. After that first successful hire, I went on to make bad hire, after bad hire, after bad hire, and it really hurt my business growth. Everything that everyone was telling me about hiring for personality, or even "experience", wasn't working.

It was out of this frustration that I decided to do something different and create what is now known across the world as **The Outcome Based Hiring System for Physical Therapists** - and subsequently wrote this book for you.

I'll be sharing the exact system that I use to hire staff at my own physical therapy practice; a system so successful that it has allowed me to go from solo practitioner – working 70 hours per week – to now having staff running my four clinics for me. Best, this allows me to spend more than 50% of my time out of the country where my practice operates.

That's right, by using the system I am about to teach you, I have built a world-class team of people that run§ my four-location clinic for me. I've got people who I can trust and this allows me to spend most of my time in another country writing books and working on a second business.

I'm living proof that if you switch your focus from hiring for personality – and even experience – to hiring for outcomes, you really can leave your clinic in the hands of people you can trust. And you can do this and still make the type of money you want without having to be there every day.

But be warned in advance: to do this right, you need to forget all of the traditional methods of hiring that you've likely come across. I get the premise of hiring for personality, but it is fundamentally flawed. Without considering what this person really needs to do for you – and if they can demonstrate proof of achieving it – you'll always make bad hires.

As I always say, <u>a wonderful personality does not come in handy when there's no money in the bank to meet payroll.</u>

To emphasize the point; imagine a situation where your favorite baseball team is recruiting for players having come off the back of a bad season. Do you think the conversation between coach and general manager is going to be about finding people with better personalities? This way of thinking would assume that all of the team's problems would be solved once they find a pitcher who is more fun to be around each day - and is happier than the last one.

There's no way that is happening. That though, is a lot of what is going on in business these days. Owners are looking to hire their version of "A-Rod", based solely off of his charm and charisma – even his willingness to learn how to throw the ball.

But what about skill levels? How and why is that being overlooked? You can spend all day, every day for five years throwing a baseball at me but I'm never developing the swinging skill needed to be a professional MLB player.

The same is true of people in business. Not all skills can be learned. Sure, some can, but not all. And that is why you should never assume that just because someone has a great personality, they'll turn out to be a hall of famer!

To compound the problem, most clinic owners do not even know what skills they're looking for let alone what outcomes they need achieving in their business. They know a great personality when they see one but they don't know how to differentiate between skills and features or indeed, how to turn tasks into quantifiable outcomes that when measured lead to better results, and higher profits.

That is what we will be putting right in the pages of this book.

You'll learn that there's a big difference between "working hard" and achieving a specific outcome, such as, for example, improving your clinics arrival rate or completed plans of care.

You'll stop thinking that just because someone comes in with a good resume, or has experience, that they're right for your role. Likewise, you'll also learn how to spot people with no experience who are right for your role.

You'll learn how to identify your major outcomes for each role – and hire people skilled enough to achieve them for you. What is more, you'll learn how to ask the right questions of candidates that reveal proof that they share your values and can actually perform as you need.

SO, WHO ARE THE RIGHT PEOPLE FOR YOUR COMPANY?

Here's the key premise of this book:

Focusing on hiring for personality should never supersede your focus on hiring someone who has the skills to solve a problem in your business.

The employees you are looking for are people with the skills to solve the problems your business has who also **share your company's values.**

It has nothing whatsoever to do with personality.

When you hire a new employee, you are entering into a relationship with that person - and them with you. Think about why most relationships breakdown; it is usually because of a lack of shared values. There's opposing differences on major things that cause a toxic or volatile relationship.

It is the same in the employee/employer relationship. After all, the reason for hiring – i.e. to solve a business problem – is rarely the reason for firing. The latter nearly always happens because of a difference of values, such as, being unwilling to learn something new, little if any consideration to time keeping or a lack of anticipating the needs of other members of staff.

A resistance to want to do these things exposes what the employee values (or doesn't!) and I believe that when people talk about hiring for personality, what they really mean is consider the *values* of the person.

The difference is profound and yet sadly, it is often lost in translation leading to a lot of heartache for clinic owners.

Hiring someone with the right skills who shares your values is not that difficult. The two are not mutually exclusive. With the right process, it is possible to find one with the other. But here's the caveat; to do so requires you to know precisely why you're hiring in the first place. As in, <u>what's the problem in your business that you need solving?</u>

Think about it... when you know what the problem is, you can look for the skills to solve that specific problem to make your business better and more profitable. But if you don't know what the real problem is, how can you look for someone appropriately skilled to solve it? You can't. And that's the problem.

I'll tell you what most do in this situation – they default to hiring for experience. The hope is that if you hire someone with experience in the role then they'll know how to do something that you can't quite articulate – but you know/feel needs doing.

Said differently, most employers resort to experience when they don't really know what they are looking for in a candidate.

But just because someone is experienced, it doesn't automatically mean they can do what you need. Experience tells you that they could hold a job down for someone else – it doesn't instantly mean they can do a good job for you. What if the thing they're good at or experienced in doing, isn't what you specifically need?

Hiring people based *solely* upon experience and personality sounds nice in theory, but in reality, it leaves many business owners with employees who start as great "culture fits" but soon end up as liabilities unable to do the job that is required.

Having the most experience or the best personality doesn't automatically make someone a great front desk person or physical therapist for your clinic. It has to be about identifying what your business' problem is – and then looking for people with the best skills to solve it (…who happen to have a nice personality).

Over the years, I've moved firmly away from hiring based on personality to what I call "hiring for outcomes", and since I've done so, the quality and strength of my employees has increased significantly. It is also no coincidence that I've experienced more growth, more profit, and more lifestyle success in that same time.

My Outcome-Based Hiring model involves four key stages:

1. **Outcome** (What problem is being solved?)

2. **Tasks** (That are needed to solve the problem)

3. **Skills** (That are required to achieve the tasks)

4. **Measure** (To make sure that the outcomes are being achieved)

All of these make up what I called the Outcomes Based Hiring Triangle:

FIG.1

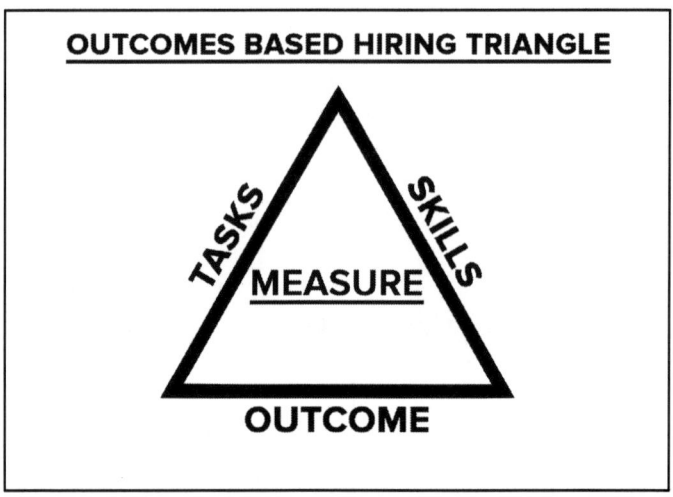

You'll see that the triangle is centered around measurement and outcomes. That is a vital component to hiring and this is because the no.1 secret to having staff that you can trust is to hold them accountable. It requires you to hire people who love to be kept accountable and then have a system to measure their results regularly.

THE ONLY TWO REASONS YOU SHOULD HIRE ANYONE

To be clear, I am not suggesting that personality and being a great cultural fit are not important – they are. It's just that there's so much focus on those things these days that business owners are becoming confused with what they are actually hiring for. So, let's clear that up now; when all is said and done, the only reason you should be hiring anyone is to **solve a business problem**. Hiring is about fulfilling a business need and, as a general rule, there are only ever really two needs in your business:

1. Getting Patients (acquisition)

2. Keeping Patients (retention)

Think about it: right now your problem is that you either can't get enough patients, or you can't keep enough patients. It is a simplistic look at the purpose of hiring, but it allows you to really narrow your focus onto why you're hiring. When you think about this, it means anyone who you employ at your clinic must be doing one of those two things or they are not required.

And what's more, they must actually be capable of doing one of those two things.

People cannot be employed just because they are a good cultural fit or even a "hard worker". Don't confuse hard workers with people who produce. The two are not the same. Seriously, if all you can say about your employees is that they are hardworking then it is a sign of a lack of accountability – on your part.

If you are not measuring the performance then there's no way of knowing what that person actually produces day-in and day-out for you. That's how you end up with a team full of underperformers who you wish you had never let step one foot inside your clinic.

Now the reason there's often no measuring of performance is nearly always because the outcomes were not clearly defined at the beginning by the owner. Most people are hired when the owner of the business feels as though they're busy enough to warrant it. It's an emotional decision caused by stuff that needs to get done, repeatedly not getting done. The owner needs help with answering the phone or sending out bills, so they hire someone to do that; to answer the phone and send out bills.

But just because they're answering the phone or mailing things out – how do you know an outcome is being achieved?

Sure, they might answer the phone by the third ring, but do they convert people into paying patients? Surely that's what you really wanted them to do, right?

And yes, they might send out the bill - but are you getting 99% of your claims settled correctly, and on time, the first time? It is one thing if the envelope goes to the local mailbox, but it is another thing entirely for what's sent to be correct. Surely, that's what you *really* wanted them to do, right?

If you don't measure these things you'll never know, and you'll end up with what I call an "office full of ants" - a place where everyone is busy being busy. There's lots of stuff getting done but when it comes to the end of the month, the profit isn't there.

To stop this, it starts by clarifying what the outcome required of your employees is and then holding them accountable to it throughout the course of their employment. This is something that we will cover in-depth in this book.

WHAT IS THE <u>OUTCOME</u> REQUIRED BY YOUR EMPLOYEES?

Primarily, this book is going to switch your focus from "do I like this person", to "can this person <u>achieve an outcome</u> that justifies the expense I have to pay for them".

Outcomes are simply problems solved. So, you need to get clear on what problems your employees solve for you.

For example, if it is a front desk person you are thinking of hiring, you need to decide if they are solving a new patient **acquisition** problem (because your inquiries don't convert), or you have a problem with drop-offs or cancels. If it is the latter, you need someone to help you solve a **retention** problem. The skills needed to achieve those outcomes are very different.

In my clinic, I have more than one person dedicated to both. That means I have someone in my admin team skilled at **acquiring** and someone skilled at **retention**. I need both, because I cannot expect the traditional "meet and greet" front of house person (that person you'll meet when you walk into most clinics) to be the one converting all of the cold leads that my direct marketing brings in. (*I showcase my entire process for bringing leads into my clinic in my first book 'New Patient Accelerator Method'*).

As we move through this book together, you will discover that it is one thing to have the skill to schedule a patient who comes to you via word of mouth or from a doctor; those patients already have some level of trust when choosing you, so they're easy to schedule. However, it is another thing entirely to be able to schedule a new patient who comes to you from a Google Ad, a Facebook or newspaper ad, or any other type of direct marketing you *should* be doing to grow your clinic actively.

Those "different" types of patients, and their current willingness to buy from you, are worlds apart. What makes them different is the point at which they are on in their buying journey and as such they require very different conversations in order to move them onto the next step.

Communication is a skill, and just like the fact that all patients aren't created equally, neither are all front desk people. They don't all have the ability to handle price objections, or to talk to cold leads who are at first, unwilling to commit to paying for physical therapy.

I can tell you from experience (both my own and the hundreds of clinic owners that I work with), that the traditional front desk person cannot do the cold lead conversion thing effectively. They are just not comfortable doing it, nor do they want to do it. They do not enjoy having conversations with cold, skeptical, and anxious patients – a process that you traditionally acquire from direct to public marketing.

The problem is this: in today's healthcare economy, you need to be able to convert the cold leads in order to grow your clinic beyond relying on word of mouth or referrals from doctors.

If you can't reach out to the public and grow your patient database proactively, then you're going to get stuck. Most clinic owners get stuck after about two years of opening, and sadly, they stay at the same level for another twenty. That's because they never master the ability to acquire and then convert cold/skeptical leads. They choose to let Sally, the traditional front of house person, try to do the clinics social media and then convert any inquires generated from it. She tries for a while and eventually fails miserably at it and yet she should never be doing either in the first place; she hasn't got the skills.

If you're getting inquires late at night on your website, or people requesting free reports from your ads on Facebook, that is great. Your marketing is working well. But, how do those same people react when they hear that they have to pay $200 in cash, or $75 copay per session (for 10 sessions) to receive the service you provide? You're going to have to do a very good job of selling the value. It can be done - but only by the right person with the right skills to do it.

If they don't have the skills then there's no way the patient will convert, and so the outcome (of getting new patients) will never be achieved.

In my clinic, the traditional front of house person is there to have fun with existing patients, to put them at ease, answer questions, and do the everyday admin stuff that keeps the clinic running. They are there to keep patients coming back (retention). They are not dealing with objections from patients having to pay huge sums of money that are incurred with copay or deductibles. I have someone in a very different seat in my clinic doing that.

This is just one example of why you've got to get clear on what it is that you're hiring for. Ask yourself, what is the real problem in your business? And it's not that you're busy! That is a symptom of being in-appropriately staffed or the ones you've got being in-efficient.

ROUND PEGS IN SQUARE HOLES

Many clinics are trying to hire round pegs and place them into square holes. The root cause of the problem is a lack of understanding of what the real problems are in the business. You can always spot when a clinic owner has hired a round peg for a square hole; they hire someone for admin tasks, and three weeks later fire them because lead conversion was down.

That is like me hiring you to be a goalkeeper for my soccer team, but later firing you because you didn't score goals! It's madness.

Another example of hiring for the wrong outcome is in the role of a physical therapist. It is widely assumed that the physical therapist should be the one who is responsible for finding their own patients. So, as well as providing a clinically excellent service, they also need to be skilled at new patient acquisition. In other words, at marketing.

Really? How is that even possible? They've spent five years studying the anatomy and physiology of the human body and now you want them to be skilled at marketing and sales? Again, this is like asking a goalkeeper in soccer to play striker. It's not going to end well. Your physical therapists are in **retention mode**. It is the job of your marketing and sales system to acquire new patients for you – and it is the job of your physical therapist to retain that patient.

Once you know what problem the physical therapist solves, it becomes much easier to hire them; it means that during the hiring process you're able to look for signs, skills – proof – that the person you're hiring is able to do to what you need them to do, that is, retain patients for you. Have they done it in the past? Do they even know or understand what their real job is?

As I said earlier, when you know what you need, you can look for it in the person you're interviewing. Coming up with questions becomes easier and from then on filling the role with the right person is all but guaranteed.

All of this and more will be covered in more depth as we move through the book together. What I'm doing in this first chapter is helping you see why hiring brings so much heartache to so many business owners; it's because they're focusing on personalities and experience, failing to consider the problem that needs solving in their business.

It is not because "it's so difficult to get good staff these days" (they were saying that 20-30 years ago as well), it's because there's no understanding of the outcome that is required. If you don't know the outcome you want, then you can't hire for the skills you need to solve the problems you've got.

If you can't solve problems, you get stuck. Personalities don't solve problems – only skills do. What is more, when you hire people to do jobs that they're actually competent in, it is amazing how the better side of their personality comes out. Just a thought.

I'VE HIRED OVER 70 STAFF – SOME HAVE BEEN WITH ME FOR ALMOST 10 YEARS

If you only read to this point in the book and no more, I want you to know that just by knowing what the outcomes of the major roles in your clinic are, you are already lightyears ahead of 99% of the physical therapy profession.

<u>You must never forget that, first and foremost, employees are hired to solve problems</u>.

At the time of writing this book, I have recruited and subsequently employed well over 70 people, in three different businesses, in two different countries. I currently employ 28 people across my different businesses – most of them in my physical therapy clinic, and that means I have lost or fired close to fifty others. I have staff members that have been with me for close to ten years, and many of them have been with me for more than five. Equally, I have staff that have come and gone – walked and pushed – in less than 7 days.

What does that mean to you? It means that I have made a lot of mistakes and subsequently learned a lot of lessons about hiring world-class people that you can trust.

As I write this to you, I have what I believe to be the strongest team that I have ever created across my group of businesses, and that is because of the hiring process that I am going to share with you in this book. It also means that everything I am sharing with you in the pages of this book is tried and true. It is a field report and not theory. It's not something that worked 10 years ago, it's what's working in physical therapy clinics around the world, and most importantly – it's what is working today.

I know what it's like to make the mistake of hiring the first candidate who arrived on time, smiled politely at me, and instantly had me thinking that this person is "the one" I've been looking for (…made easier to hire because the other person didn't show up). I know what it is like to take too long to get my butt into gear to start the hiring process and then subsequently rush the decision – one that I would later come to regret.

But, I have since been able to create a predictable and repeatable system that has served me well across three businesses and in two different countries. I have been able to create a system for recruiting people with the right skills to solve specific problems in my business; people who enjoy the fact that I call it tight, talk straight, and know that I am holding them accountable for achieving the outcome for which they were employed.

You could say that, in over a decade of recruiting people, I've learned that almost **everything I was ever taught about hiring was wrong**.

Ultimately, I've learned that hiring people solely for personality is what gets you into trouble. If you want to be able to hire great people that you can trust (so that you can take more than one day off without worrying or being called in to solve a problem created in your absence), then you have to recruit people who have skills to solve your problems and who love achieving outcomes; people that also share your company values.

To be able to trust people you have to inspect what they are doing. And to be able to do that you have employ people who are happy to be held accountable for achieving outcomes in the first place. That requires you to know what those outcomes look like, and that is why measuring is vital to your success.

The right person recognizes that far from "spying" on what they are doing, assuming that you're looking for another excuse to criticize a weakness, you are actually looking for clues as to where their performance is currently off so that you can help them.

Do you see the difference?

Of course, those same people are going to be hired with the values that makes them likely to be a great culture fit, but they are not being hired solely because they have a great personality.

That is the big difference I am going to teach you and when you switch your clinics hiring to the outcomes-based model that I am presenting, it will be liberating for you; best it will show in your profit and lifestyle account.

Not only will you be clearer on who you are hiring – you'll also be clearer on what they are actually doing for you. With that, you'll know what to do to step in and help them make improvements to their performance as it is needed. When you do that, your company will go from **high maintenance to high performance**.

If that is what you want, let's move into chapter 2, where I'll tell you a true story of the biggest hiring mistake I ever made…

2

THE BIGGEST HIRING MISTAKE I EVER MADE (THAT COST ME $100,000'S...)

One of the biggest mistakes you can make in your hiring is to hire from your "gut" or "emotion". It might feel nice at the time, but it's not long before you realize that your gut gets you into trouble. Other than when I am hungry, I don't rely on it all that much these days. And yet it hasn't always been that way... I'd go so far as to say that hiring on gut or emotion is perhaps the biggest hiring mistake I've ever made. I learned this lesson the very hard way right after I employed my first full time employee Vicki Smith.

True story: Vicki was a former patient, recommended to me by a mutual friend. I didn't know her at all before she came in to the clinic, but when she arrived for her first appointment I knew that there was something different about her.

She just had something – I could feel it in my "gut".

She had the type of people skills and personality that you could only dream of being around each day. After a few sessions working on her shoulder, I had a great "feeling" (in my gut again) that she would be the perfect person to solve the front desk issue I had at the time.

The issue I had at the time was this: I didn't have anyone at my front desk and I needed someone.
The phone was ringing and no one was answering it. I was busy treating patients, and that meant I was losing patients (retention

problem). People wanted to hire me, but I couldn't get them on schedule because I was too busy treating those already on the schedule. I couldn't be in two places at once.

Towards the end of her treatment I asked Vicki about her employment situation. She said she wasn't overly happy at work, and so it was the perfect match; I had a job – and she didn't want the one she currently had.

Vicki turned out to be the perfect person to do the job. Nearly ten years later and she is still with me. I landed a real superstar and I didn't even have to go through any formal hiring process. I thought all hiring worked like this. And because of my early success, I thought all hiring functioned this way, but I was about to learn a very hard lesson…

I'd love to write and tell you that I hired this superstar based off of the world-class outcome-based hiring process I am sharing with you now. But, I didn't. I winged it. I literally struck gold! I didn't even have to buy a ticket and I won the lottery that day.

In reality, all that happened was I got the right side of the 50-50 decision that could have gone horribly wrong.

But, what followed was a series of bad (and some very bad) hires that all arrived at my practice under the same process as the one Vicki had arrived by. They didn't all start as patients with a supraspinatus tear in their shoulder, but they were each hired with the same type of process and logic as Vicki. Which was basically this: "you seem like a nice person; do you want a job?"

Back then, all you had to do was smile at me and tell a story about you helping an old lady across the road and I'd have given you a job!

My recruitment "process" even extended to asking Vicki, "who do you know?", and then giving one or two people a job just because they were friends or family of Vicki's.

My logic was this: Vicki is a nice person and is good at what she does. Vicki has shown me that nice people are good at this job. If I just find more nice people like Vicki, I'll get more people good at their job! Anyone who hangs around with Vicki must be a nice person.

It appeared that all I had to do was ask, "Vicki, who do you know that wants a job?"

It's laughable to me today, but that is how I operated back then and it's how many still operate today. My results? I had a lot of "nice" people in my practice, but I didn't always have employees who were able to achieve my results. Two and two didn't always equal four, and when it got to the point of me having to fire one of Vicki's family members, I realized that my recruitment process was flawed… and if I fired another member of her family, it wouldn't be long before she quit.

After hiring Vicki and getting that decision right, I think the next three employees came and went very quickly. As I look back, it was obvious why: I had used the same process as I did to hire Vicki, that is, I assumed that my gut knows best. Turns out it doesn't. The success of Vicki just made me stupid and cost me a lot of money, hours, and training, all of which were lost to the procession of bad hires that followed.

As I look back at the reason why Vicki did last the course with me (ten years plus and counting), I know now it wasn't *just* because of her great personality. It was because she had previously worked in a similar role at a dental clinic. She had already done things like coding (ICD 10 equivalent), billing insurance, and upselling dental patients to the hygienist – all I had to do was teach her the difference between what they say at the dentist and what we do in physical therapy.

Guess what that meant for me? That's right, she already had the <u>skills</u> needed to do the job. That meant all I had to do was optimize those skills for my clinic. I wasn't starting from scratch with someone who had no level of training. Which meant she was able to solve my problems immediately and without too much fuss.

Vicki arrived as a very good employee – and I believe to this day she is truly world-class. There isn't a person on earth, not anywhere that I've been, who I would trade her for. She is *that* good. I hired her for personality – and luckily for me she had the skills that I could work with and improve.

I believe that the combination of her initial skill set, plus my coaching and optimizing her for a physical therapy clinic, is why she not only lasted, but has also excelled beyond my wildest dreams.

The three employees that followed all had the personality, but not the skills. I could not train the skill. They did not last. In Vicki's case I was optimizing the skill already there. But, I didn't have to teach her how to do it from scratch. That is huge for you to understand.

I see a lot of clinic owners looking for "experience" in the exact same role as they're advertising. But that is not what you need to look for; you need to find people who have used the skills you need in your role. In Vicki's case, she'd already been developing the skills that I was looking for, at the dentist. It made it more likely she would be a success for me.

I got lucky with Vicki. My ignorance was bliss and I got away with it, but I paid the price with the next three. Do not copy me. What you need is a hiring process that delivers data on candidates based upon their history, allowing you to create a profile of them. Doing this moves the odds from 50-50, to **80-20**, and obviously gives you a significantly higher chance of getting this right more times than not. You'll get that process from this book.

Hiring from gut and emotion is just one of the many mistakes that leads to the types of hires that give you sleepless nights and endless headaches. Let's take a look at a few more of the common ones. By cutting out the things that land you with bad hires, you'll get closer to the great hires that you want.

RECRUITMENT MISTAKE #2 – THINKING A "CRAPPY 3 LINE AD ON CRAIG'S LIST" WOULD ATTRACT QUALITY CANDIDATES!

In my first book, *"The New Patient Accelerator Method"*, (available at www.PaulsMarketingBook.com), I dedicated much of the text to the importance of using your marketing to identify the right "target market" (the perfect patient) for your clinic. Well, it is the same with recruitment; you have to use your marketing skills to attract the right person in order to solve the problems you have.

Putting out a job description and suggesting your role is suitable for anyone and everyone, is a mistake. Doing so is going to have you inundated with applications from anyone – from pizza delivery drivers to janitors – all looking for a job! That is fine, and there's nothing wrong with either of those roles, but I am pretty sure that neither will have the skills you need to acquire or retain patients for your physical therapy clinic.

A lack of marketing for the position and really selling the role to the right person, allows everyone who sees the ad it to think that they are qualified for it and should apply for the job you're recruiting for. And many do. You are flattered by the response - but you're now overwhelmed with candidates all desperate for a job. And with 100 random applications to go through for your role, what chance have you got of getting it right? The odds are slim.

Imagine what it would be like if you only had to go through 10 applications and all 10 of those were ideal candidates. You'd have so much more time to dedicate to the candidate, asking more questions and thinking long and hard about your decision. The odds of getting it right have already swung in your favor, and that situation is possible with the system I am outlining in this book.

So, even with recruitment you have to follow the timeless rules of marketing: repel and attract. Repel the people you do not want and attract the people you do want. Do this by using your job advert to talk about the skills required, and even politely tell people not to apply unless they have a proven track record of using those skills to solve the problems you need them to. (In chapter 8, we will go through exactly how you create ads like this.)

RECRUITMENT MISTAKE #3 – PICKING THE BEST OF A BAD BUNCH

Most people arrive at their new position by default; they are only given the job because the other candidates where so **underwhelming** it made them out to be "rock stars", despite the obvious limitations.

The one other guy who was scheduled for an interview arrived late, so he got ruled out. Sarah, the one who arrived five minutes early, instantly gets the job because it is now seemingly "obvious" she is "committed" and really wants the job. After all, she did arrive five minutes early, which *proves* the theory. The fact that Sarah arrived five minutes early for an interview is great, but what about her ability to solve the problem she is being hired to do? Does she even know how to answer the phone?

To avoid this problem, you need what I call **"deal flow"** – a supply of quality candidates, all of whom call you to have a sleepless night because you don't know which one you will choose. It is only when you get to this point that you should be making a decision. If you don't get to this point – start again.

How do you get deal flow? By positing your job on more than just Craig's List or Indeed. In chapter 9, I'll share with you more than ten places you could, and should, place your job posting ads.

RECRUITMENT MISTAKE #4 – HIRING BASED OFF OF A FAMILY, OR FRIENDS, RECOMMENDATION

It is one thing to use your close circle of friends, family, and even current employees to ask if they know anyone who might actively be seeking employment. But, it is something else entirely to hire them based solely off of the same recommendation.

It is ok to entertain the person as a possibility, but just because they came highly recommended, does not mean they're the right person to do your job. Nobody knows what you need better than you. They may have been the right person in another environment for someone else, or for another position, but how does that automatically mean they're going to be great for you?

Some of my early hiring nightmares came because I accepted the recommendation of family members. I was assured that they could vouch for the person they were recommending. The problem I later recognized was this: they were vouching for something I was not looking for.

Almost every time a friend or family member recommended someone to me, they were doing so because the person was "trustworthy, honest and reliable" – even "great" at what they do. And it turns out they were great… just not at doing the job that I needed doing.

Retrospectively, I look at those early hiring situations and realize the reason I accepted such recommendations was because I was fearful of the hiring process; I had no clue how to do it, and it became easier just to hire someone's friend or relative.

Not only was I fearful of the process, I was worried about who I could trust. I had heard the horror stories about embezzlement; I knew that we had cash on premises, and it was overwhelming to try and hire a stranger not knowing if I could trust them. I was an early business owner stepping my toes into the murky water of employment. I was looking more to protect myself from the consequences of getting hiring wrong than I was about finding a strong candidate.

I thought that by hiring on a friend or family member's recommendation, I would be able to trust them.

At that time, I was using 'not stealing from me' as my only metric of success. Meaning, if the person I hired did not help themselves to the money in my till en-route to Starbucks, then I had hired a winner!

Here's the thing: they didn't do me any harm in the sense of robbing or stealing from me, and they did show up for work on time each day. Yes, they were great at that, but they couldn't do what I needed to get done. In fact, I sometimes wish they had stolen from me because I'd have been able to get rid of them quicker. It would have cost me less than their poor performance was costing me each day.

Use a friend or family member's understanding of the person's qualities to validate the decision you have already made once they have been through your full process – but do not make it solely off what they say.

RECRUITMENT MISTAKE #5 – NOT HIRING AT ALL

People will do anything to avoid hiring. And I understand why: it is because it is so episodic. You do it so infrequently that you don't get the chance to be great at it.

The irony is that you get better at it the more you do it. But, you don't get the chance to get better at it until your clinic is growing. And yet, you're only going to grow if you hire the right people. It is a closed loop of success that, once you get there, allows you to grow faster in one year than you did in the first ten. On the next page I'll show you how it looks…

FIG.2 – CLOSED LOOP OF HIRING SUCCESS AND BUSINESS GROWTH

HIRE RIGHT PEOPLE → GROW → HIRE MORE RIGHT PEOPLE → MORE GROWTH →

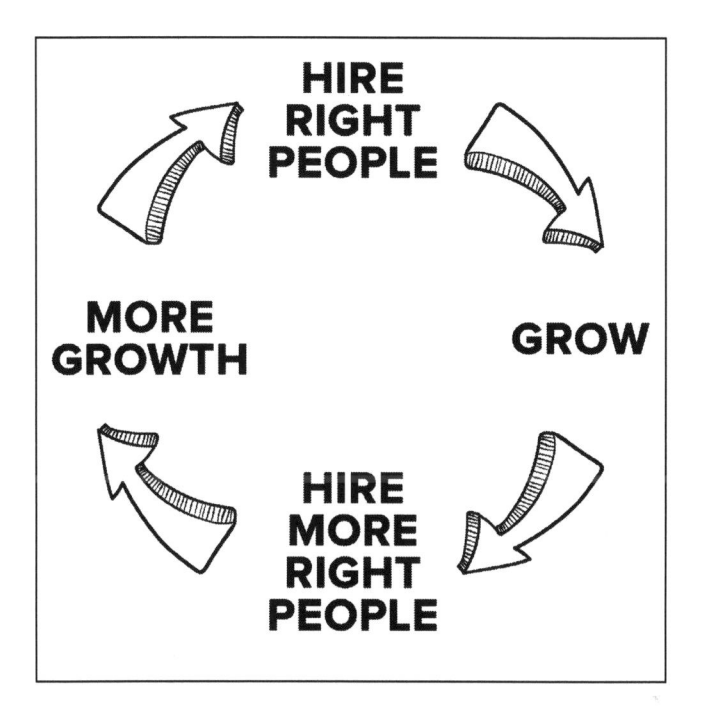

EMPLOYEES COME WITH A PAYMENT PLAN

The other reason people shy away from hiring is because they assume they're in line to deal with all sorts of legal issues and consequences if they get it wrong. Or, they fear being lumbered with an employee that they can't pay for if business drops. I understand that; but, never forget that **employees come with a payment plan**.

And, you can stop that payment plan after 90 days if it doesn't work out. You can often do this without any legal come back, as long as the contract of employment is done right. (Of course, I am not a lawyer, and employment laws vary from state to state and country-to-country, therefore I recommend you check with your own lawyer or attorney to be accurate on this – but for the most part, it's possible).

If you're nervous about hiring, it's a sign that you're not sure on the outcome. When you are clear about the outcome it is easy to tie those outcomes to actual dollar figures. This all but ensures that your new employee will actually pay for themselves. It's like a guarantee that you can't lose money. After a set period of time (i.e. 90 days), either they are <u>keeping your patients</u> or they are <u>getting you more patients.</u>

If they do the job they were hired for, how can you not afford to pay for them? And on the contrary, if people are not hitting the objectives you agreed at the outset of the employment, you let them go. It is that simple.

RECRUITMENT MISTAKE #6 – WAITING TOO LONG TO BE "READY"

Most people wait too long to recognize that they need to hire. By the time they have recognized the need, they are desperate for the help. This leads to poor hiring decisions, no time to create a plan (discussed in Chapter 5) and hiring too fast. It is a catastrophic position to be in when hiring.

If hiring is not part of a plan you've set for your business, then you'll be doing it because you desperately need help. Or, alternately, you'll be reacting to another resignation you didn't see coming.

When you let it go too long, your better judgment will be clouded by the pain of whatever is happening in your business. You know that it's past the point of needing someone to answer the phone. You're now trying to juggle your role as a physical therapist (and business owner) with more on your plate than one person can even handle. And of course, you've just made the load even worse by taking on the role of a full-time recruiter.

In this time-crunched situation, something has to give. And it's usually the recruitment process that falls by the way side. Taking care of business is more important than taking time to save time, and the hiring decision is then often rushed. When you end up in this position your chances of success are slim to none.

There's a fine line between deciding to hire in advance of a business need and waiting until the need is obvious or pressing. If you choose the latter, it's likely that the only problem that you will be solving is the problem that feeling like you need to hire creates!

RECRUITMENT MISTAKE #7 – TRUSTING A RESUME

There's so much emphasis placed upon a person's "resume", but truth be told, I tend to ignore it.

The resume tells you things like where the person was educated at, what jobs they've held in the past, and the qualifications received at school. And doesn't it always look great? So great, in fact, that it's tempting to let the resume make the decision for you.

However, it is said that something like 70% of resumes contain false information – only you have no way of knowing which parts true, and which parts are fabrications of the truth.

Some of my worst employees had the best resumes, and after making the mistake of letting a resume cloud my judgment once too often, I decided to flip the way that I use it; I now use the resume retrospectively (after the first interview). I use it to validate the decision I am about to make. I prefer to read it after an interview so that I am not in any way biased or blinded by how well the person is trying to convince me of the things they want me to believe about them.

Really, all I want to know is, can you solve the problem that I've got? And if so, then I want to know if your values match up to mine. I'll ask them the questions in the interview that I believe are appropriate to the role –and then I'll cross check what they have told me with their resume later on. (I go through the questions I use in chapter 10).

Now, don't get me wrong on this, the resume is important, but I've come to look at the resume as a something that gets them to the interview – it does not get them the job. Big difference.

RECRUITMENT MISTAKE #8 – THINKING THAT THEY ACTUALLY WANT THE JOB THEY ARE APPLYING FOR

It is said that something like 71% of all people in a job right now are dis-satisfied. That means they don't necessarily want the job you are offering – they just don't want the job that they currently have.

I've experienced at least a dozen occasions over the years when I've interviewed someone for a role who has told me, to my face, that what I am offering is their "dream job". And yet, when I offered it to them, they "regret to inform me that they need to decline my offer."

For example, one of the biggest challenges I have, as an employer in the private healthcare sector in the UK, is the free socialist system. It not only makes it tough to convince patients to pay me cash out of pocket (for a service that is available free, paid for by the government), but it also makes it difficult to attract employees.

It is almost impossible for a small company like mine to offer people the same type of benefits they get from a government-based health care system; these benefits might include six weeks paid vacation, flexi-time (start and finish when you want), nine months paid maternity, twelve months of sick pay, significant pension contributions, and so on. All of this combined means that, although they may not be overly happy in their current career working in the system, it makes coming into the private sector to work for me a much bigger decision.

When people apply for jobs at my clinic they know their benefits will never be as robust as the government's. But, at the time of applying, their dis-satisfaction with their career causes them to feel like they're happy to give those benefits all up in search of a better, more rewarding career in the private sector – in which, by the way, they will actually be able to make more money, albeit with a little less security.

Their unhappiness at work clouds their judgment, and they tell themselves they can live without those benefits. But, when they actually get offered the job, a discussion takes place at home later that night between them and their husband, wife, or partner, (sometimes even mother and father), and instead of being about what they might gain from the job, they start focusing on what they will lose. They then get cold feet and reconsider their decision.

This is important for you to understand; as a general rule, people will always choose unhappiness over uncertainty. Meaning, people can, and will, live with being unhappy because they know what they're getting – even if it isn't great. But, ask them to do something <u>uncertain</u> and they'll not want to do it for fear of it being even worse.

This is a fundamental law of human behavior, and as you're managing or leading people it is helpful to understand things like this.

The first couple of times this happened to me it infuriated me! I used to take it personally. I used to think that people were wasting my time. That was until I realized exactly what was going on; they didn't always want my job, they just didn't want their current job.

Knowing this, I made two significant changes to my hiring process: I made sure to have that deal flow I spoke about earlier, which is achieved by having a process that identifies at least three solid candidates for every role. When/if the one that I offer the role to goes back to their current employer and uses my job offer to hold them to ransom for improved conditions, I am not phased if they then later tell me thanks, but no thanks.

"BEFORE YOU ACCEPT, DO YOUR HOMEWORK ON ME!"

The second change that I made involves when, and how, I actually offer any jobs; I have stopped giving people the job outright.

Here's what I do instead: I tell them that they are the one that I want to hire. But, I also tell them that I want them to go away and first do their homework on *me* before they say yes.

I stop them from accepting the job for at least 48 hours after I offer it. And in that time, I tell them to do more research on *me*.

I tell them to ask anyone and everyone they know for information on me; to look on social media channels, search me on the internet, and literally try and dig up anything that they can about me that would stop them from wanting to come and work for me.

This has been a huge game changer for me. The level of confidence it takes to tell someone to go away and dig for information on you is stunning. It is sending an instant message to the person that you've got in front of you that you have nothing to hide. There are no skeletons in the closet. There'll be no unexpected surprises waiting for them when they get here.

This final part of the process helps dampen any worries of an employee coming from a big company, where they assume they're going to be "safer" and in a job for "life", to a small company like yours and mine where other people will assume there is more risk.

Asking potential employees to do their homework on you before accepting your offer mitigates this, and has employees arriving a lot more confident than before I did it. This also gives me 48 hours of breathing space before I tell the other people they didn't get the role, people who, in fact, I might still need to go to!

There are a few lessons here: if you're a small clinic owner, it pays to understand the level of risk involved in coming to work for you (over a bigger name or national chain), so that you can mitigate it. Secondly, do not get overly excited about any candidate. And equally, do not get overly disappointed or frustrated if you offer them a job that they accept and later decline.

For all of the reasons outlined above, such a reaction on the part of the candidate is perfectly normal. The solution to this is a hiring process that delivers at least 3 great candidates, putting you in a position where you are having a sleepless night over which one you are going to hire. That is because any one of them could be right for you.

RECRUITMENT MISTAKE #9 – MAKING YOUR MIND UP IN THE FIRST 5 MINUTES OF THE INTERVIEW

Statistics show that 80% of employers make up their mind in the first <u>five</u> minutes of the interview. They are "trusting their gut feeling" about what they are seeing and feeling, and they then spend the rest of the interview validating their decision. Even though there are no signs or clues that this person has ever done anything like what you need them to do for you in the past, something is telling you that they'll be able to do it for you.

Whether it is the smile, the look, their personality, or even their nodding of approval or understanding every time you tell them about your vision for your business, all of these become the "signs" that this is the right person for the job! This is madness. And yet, it is happening.

If you're a veteran employer, my bet is that you've done this more than once? If so, the key to setting yourself up for holding a successful interview is to <u>suspend your judgment for as long as possible.</u> If you're struggling with doing this, then go into the interview with a completely different perspective or way of looking at it…

Instead of asking yourself if this is the right person, look for reasons that this is the wrong person. Flip the reasoning. Ask yourself, "why should I NOT hire this person", or "why should I completely ignore this candidate?"

When you change the question, you will always change the outcome.

If by the end of the first 20 minutes you can't find any reason not to give them the job, then all that happens is that they make it to the next phase. It is a radical shift in your thinking, and if you can't help but like anyone and everyone who comes in, I recommend you try this approach.

Remember, this is the most important decision any business owner has to make. With the right people, you can solve any problem in your business. The more you solve problems, the better your business will be. It is worth focusing on protecting yourself from the evils of getting it wrong, rather than usually assuming it is always going to go right.

The same is true in life and business. Sometimes it pays to spend more time trying to avoid the big down side, rather than just chasing the good stuff all the time.

According to Warren Buffet (the world's richest investor), Rule #1 of investing is "don't lose money", and Rule #2 is "never forget rule #1". As a business owner, you are always investing: both in yourself and your business. In the case of hiring, I think that Buffet's rule could be modified to this:

Rule #1: Don't make a rash or snap decision

Rule #2: Always refer to rule #1

RECRUITMENT MISTAKE #10 – ASKING YOUR ACCOUNTANT IF YOU SHOULD HIRE

I can always spot a business owner who takes their accountant's advice; they usually have minimal staff and no marketing system. They're always tired, stressed, and overworked trying to do more than they can handle.

Think about it: accountants are paid an awful lot of money to do stuff that most business owners don't really understand. They know full well we are frustrated by having to pay their high fees, (for doing stuff that is forced upon us), and in attempt to justify those fees they'll look for ways to make us 'a bit more money'.

It makes them, and us, feel so much better about the fee we have to cough up. There are two problems with this:

1. It nearly always involves <u>cutting</u> expenses

2. An accountant's definition of expenses is flawed

Accountants consider marketing and staff as expenses. And yet any business owner trying to grow is going to need both.

Now, you can make more profit by cutting your expenses, but only to a certain point. After a while, you end up cutting so much from the day to day running of the business that there's nothing left to leverage. Without leverage, owners end up doing more than they should be, and that's why so many owners are tired and stuck. You get leverage from having staff.

What is more, staff are not expenses; they are assets. It is important to see them this way, because **income follows assets**. If you want more income, you need more assets.

Two of your best assets in business are **people,** and your **marketing system**. Coincidentally, both are nearly always the first things that any accountants want to cut from your expenses.

And I've had it happen to me. The first full time accounts person I brought into my group of companies was quite literally shell-shocked when he realized that my "bill" for marketing expenditure across my company, was well over $250,000.

He "advised" me that next year we might want to "cut that back" a little. *I* advised *him* that the only reason he was in a job was because of the income produced by that $250,000+ spend on marketing.

He not only went quiet, but he very quickly started to understand why so many of the companies that he'd worked for in the past were not able to grow. They view things such as marketing and staff as expenses – not the revenue generators that they are.

Here's a word of caution about accountants: in my experience, they want to cut so many expenses that in the end, it actually harms the business owner more than it helps.

Cutting out staff and eradicating marketing budgets – even business coaching and training – sentences the business owner to a lifetime of perpetual struggle of dependence upon him or herself doing everything. When you cut out marketing it means that there's only one way to grow - the slow and unpredictable way of relying upon word of mouth referrals. But just because they're "free" doesn't mean it is the best way.

And just because it's "free" doesn't mean it is not costing you money elsewhere.

Let me make it abundantly clear:

1. **Accountants should never be consulted for business advice** - they are there to advise you on how to keep your taxes at a legal minimum. That's it. They do not, and never will, know what it takes to grow your business. Do not be fooled by their position of authority or ever be tempted to

relegate the big decisions in your business to someone who is trained to cut expenses and file taxes.
2. **Staff are assets** - and income follows assets. If you want more income, you need more assets. The goal of a business is to turn assets, (your marketing system and staff), into revenue. Then turn that revenue into profit, (by minimizing the expense required to deliver the outcome promised by marketing), and turn that profit into cash...

...And with that cash you can do three things:

1. Pay down business debt

2. Reinvest it into the business

3. Dividend it out (i.e. take it home and spend it)

What I have just described to you is how a business works. It is the only way a business can ever work, and, if you want your business to grow, you need to start thinking less about keeping down costs and more about investing in <u>income producing assets</u>, i.e. staff and marketing.

It is about being efficient with your expenses. It is not about eradicating them completely to the point that it stops your growth. Marketing and people are dynamic expenses that should be controlled – not cut out.

Ok, so that's the most common hiring mistakes covered. Next, we're going to look at the structure of a world-class company. Before you rush out and hire the next person, it's important to consider the position that candidate will hold in your company, and furthermore, how each role you fill impacts one that you've already got filled.

Turn the page and let's get going...

@THEPAULGOUGH

3

THE STRUCTURE OF ALL WORLD-CLASS COMPANIES

Most clinic owners hire sequentially; it's a succession of admin or physical therapists coming into the clinic as the need arises. However, after a few years of doing just that - hiring people as the need becomes apparent - owners soon find themselves with a clinic that is an inefficient mess or one that has ground to a halt completely. Sound familiar?

This situation happens frequently – and largely because zero consideration has gone into the other departments that are necessary for all businesses to thrive and grow sustainably.

In this chapter I am going to explain how to avoid that happening to you. And, how to unravel it if it already has. Essentially, I am going show you how your company should be structured; where all of your employees should be positioned in relation to one another, and how they all should work together for the good of the long-term growth of your company.

To grow, your company must be the total sum of all the parts required of an organization. It can never be solely reliant upon delivering a great physical therapy service, no matter how skilled you are.

If you like, this is a higher-level look at your business. It is more strategic than just "who" or "how to hire." It is a birds-eye view of all of the roles you will need to fill as your business grows, and in this chapter, I'll also explain how all of the roles in your company are interconnected; how each person you employ impacts the next person. Think of what I am about to teach you as a map or a framework for all of your future hiring decisions. It is necessary to ensure that the next hire you make, and everyone thereafter, is the one you need and is someone who will bring the most impact to your bottom line.

INTRODUCING THE COMPANY ORGANIZATIONAL CHART

The image below is called an **org chart** (company organizational chart) and its purpose is to allow you to see the relationships of the departments - and people - in your business. An org chart can act as a guide for who you should be hiring next, and in what department.

Take a look at the image below:

FIG.3 COMPANY ORG CHART – TOP LINE DEPARTMENTS

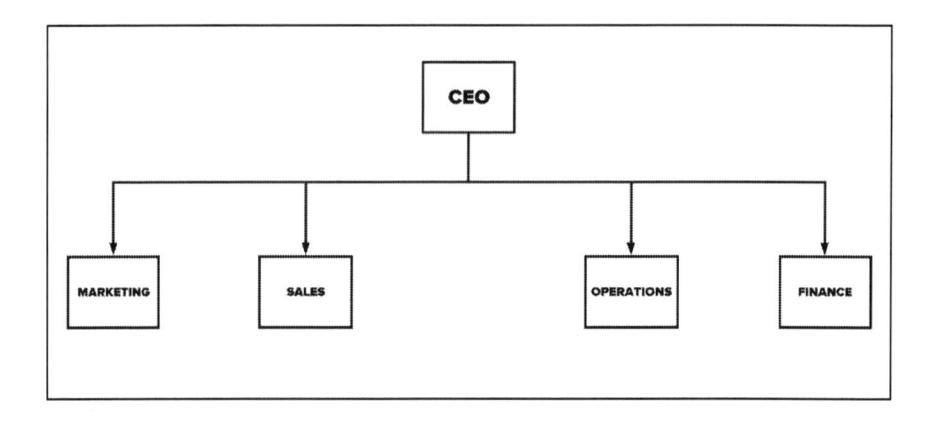

It shows four departments across the top line. That is because every successful business starts with four departments on the top line. These are your top tier staffs, sometimes known as the "Leadership Team" or "C-Level" employees (CFO, COO etc.).

It is important to understand the relationship between each one and to know that each department is connected to another; the performance of one directly affects the ability of the other. Let's look more closely at the departments:

- **Marketing** – its job is to make people aware that you exist and to show how you can solve their problems (i.e. run ads in the newspaper or on Facebook about how your clinic can help people walk without back pain).

- **Sales** – its job is to continue the conversation started by the marketing department and turn inquiries/interest into patients (i.e. convert a lead from a newspaper ad to an initial evaluation/paying patient).

- **Operations** – its job is to make good on the promise made by the sales person (i.e. the physical therapist providing the care/skills to help someone walk without back pain).

- **Finance** – its job is to collect payment once the promise has been fulfilled by the operations team (i.e. at the end of the treatment provided by the physical therapist).

The four departments are required for every business to be successful. Depending on how big you are, it could be the case that you are doing all of those things yourself right now – you just didn't know it.

If you are currently doing everything, pay close attention to this universal structure. As you begin to strip back from doing all of the activities – and you start hiring – it allows you to replace yourself accordingly. That is putting the right people in the right seats at the right time so that you as you grow, you do so with minimal hassle and maximum profitability.

As I always say, growing profitably is the goal. It is not about getting big for the sake of getting big. I know a lot of "big" clinic owners who don't make big take home pay, and that's because they flout the rules of company growth and structure.

Now, if you've already grown to a certain size, it may be the case that as you look at this org chart, you're finding that you've got the same person in three or four places. For example, your "rock star" front desk person is doing the operations stuff, the billing, and you're expecting her to do the marketing and selling too.

If that is the case, you should also be expecting her resignation imminently, as it is not possible for her to cope or perform at a high level in all those sectors.

Most clinics have their structure all wrong: there are people who should be in operations (i.e. physical therapists), but who are being expected to market and sell. Or, clinics have front desk people being expected to "do a bit of marketing" as well as provide great customer service.

The above org chart flags this up and gives you a visual of why so many physical therapy clinics struggle. It shows why there's so much inefficiency in many clinics, and ultimately, why most clinic owners end up making less than their employees. It's because there's a lack of thought going into who is hired, why and when!

THE STRUCTURE OF A CLINIC THAT IS STUCK

If you have been in business for more than five years, and let's say you've got more than ten staff, chances are your org chart looks something like the chart on the next page…

FIG.4

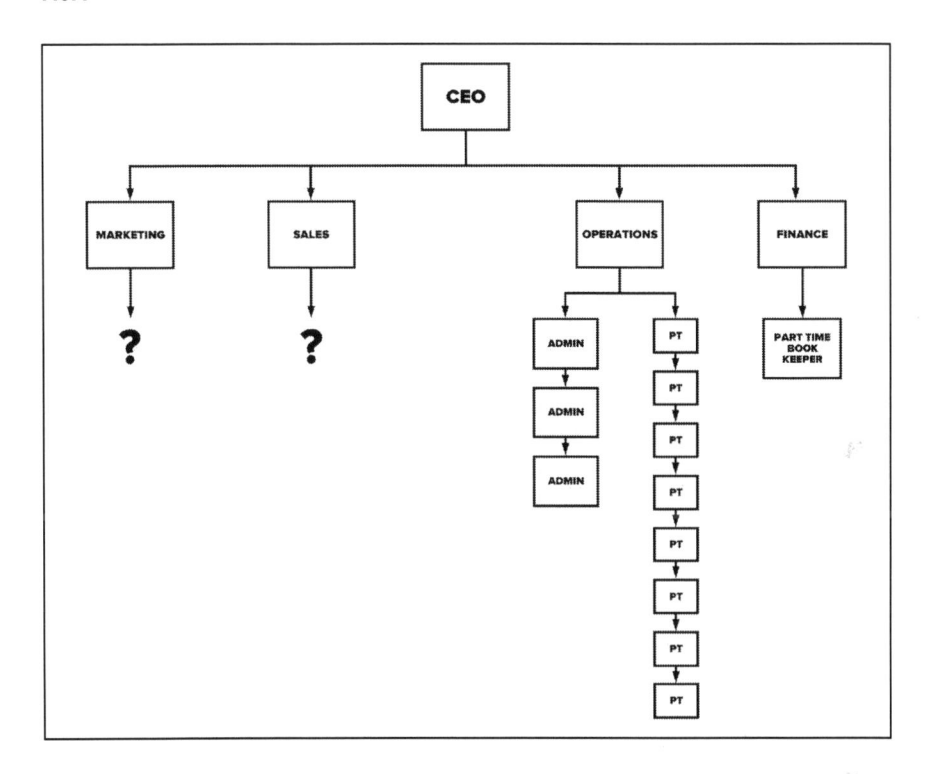

[Organizational chart showing CEO at top, with four branches: Marketing (with "?" below), Sales (with "?" below), Operations (branching into three Admin boxes and a column of eight PT boxes), and Finance (with Part Time Book Keeper below).]

It doesn't take a rocket scientist to work out that it is not propped up correctly. As you can see, the org chart is rather one sided, in fact, it is grossly "lop-sided". All of the emphasis is on delivering a service with the marketing and sales completely overlooked. This is why so many clinics get stuck. There's lots of staff waiting to deliver a great service but not enough people coming in.

With a clinic that is structured like this, the owner is essentially trying to ride a two-legged horse, yet still expecting to win the race. The operations department is full of great therapists and admin people, but there's no one looking after marketing or sales.

Please tell me, how do you keep ten therapists and admin busy if there's no one doing any marketing or selling?

THE TWO-LEGGED HORSE DOESN'T WIN MANY RACES

I remember a call I had with a clinic owner who reached out to me saying they had a "marketing problem". The owner told me that he was the one doing the marketing for the clinic, so I asked him what his commitment to marketing was. He said $2000 per month. I said no, what's your real commitment – how much <u>time</u> do you invest? He said "5-6 hours, or whenever I get chance".

Now after doing this exercise with him, I said "you do have a marketing problem - the problem is no one is doing any marketing!"

I explained that, if he simply gave the same time and commitment to marketing as he does operations, he wouldn't have a problem.

I then asked how long his clinic had been stuck for, and he said over two years. I asked why he hadn't employed a full-time marketer, and he told me it was because he couldn't afford it. Why couldn't he afford it? Because he was over staffed. He'd employed more and more admin, expecting that they'd always be able to keep growing on the word of mouth stuff that they were relying on heavily.

And, of course, he thought like most clinic owners do that one of those admin staff members would step up and take over the clinics marketing or manage the social media channels. Marketing box checked. As for sales? Well, the ignorant assumption in health care is that the service somehow sells itself and so almost everyone overlooks needing to have someone in a seat who can talk about money and overcome objections to it.

The reality is that this is how most clinics are structured and is also why they're stuck. There's no understanding of what it actually takes to grow a company that is strong and stable - one that grows efficiently and profitably.

Having five admin, five therapists, your mother-in-law doing your billing (when she gets around to it), and you as the owner doing a "bit of marketing" – likely only when your patients don't turn up – and thinking your service will sell itself – *is* the problem. It is not a lack of leads or a marketing problem that most owners think they've got – it's that the company is not structured correctly to allow it to function.

And unless (or until) you fix *that*, nothing will change.

EXERCISE: DRAW YOUR OWN COMPANY ORG CHART AS IT LOOKS TODAY

If you have already got staff, as a fun exercise, draw out the org chart for yourself and just start to put people's names in departments (…I've put some examples of an org chart in your resources PDF that accompanies this book. You can download that here: www.paulgough.com/hiring-resource).

Literally, just draw the chart out on a piece of paper and see who is where in your organization. Just put their initials in the appropriate box; see how many people are in the same place multiple times, and then ask yourself an important question:

Has the person doing all of those jobs really got the right skill set to be doing them? And, did you even know you had hired them to do be doing all of those different roles?

My bet is that for most people reading this book, once you've done that exercise you'll already start getting an idea about why your company isn't performing at the level you would like; why it is more high maintenance than high performance.

If that is the case, it's happening because you've got the wrong people in the wrong seats. Or, someone in multiple seats unable to perform tasks due to a lack of time in which to do them.

When I learned how a company must be structured (to be successful long term), it all made perfect sense why my own company was struggling, and, why I felt so stuck just a few years after starting. I was trying to grow, and yet I was ignoring the rules of how a business must be structured for growth. I was paying the price with less profit than I thought I deserved for the work I was putting in. It didn't matter how hard I worked or "hustled", it seemed that there was no real difference to the profit at the end of the month.

It was happening because I was guilty of putting the wrong people in the wrong roles, oblivious to how they are all supposed to work in tandem.

That's why I want to bring this to your attention early on in the book. There's no point in having a great hiring process if you're hiring the wrong people at the wrong time or for the wrong role. All that happens is that you end up with more people than you need and less profit than you want. That's not what I want for you.

HOW THE FOUR DEPARTMENTS WORK TOGETHER

So, with that in mind, let me explain how all four departments work together. Here is the image of top line of the org chart displayed for you to look at again:

FIG.5

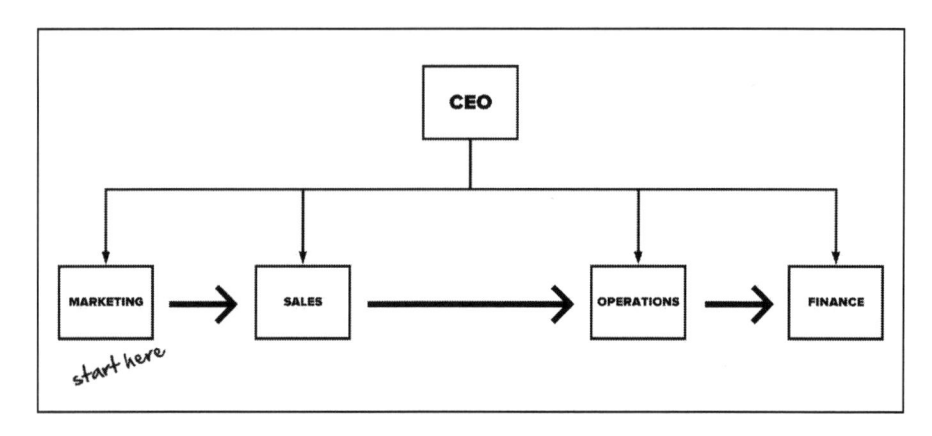

```
                    ┌─────┐
                    │ CEO │
                    └──┬──┘
        ┌──────────┬───┴────┬──────────┐
        ▼          ▼        ▼          ▼
   ┌─────────┐ ┌─────┐ ┌──────────┐ ┌────────┐
   │MARKETING│→│SALES│→│OPERATIONS│→│FINANCE │
   └─────────┘ └─────┘ └──────────┘ └────────┘
   start here
```

You'll see the four departments from left to right; the order in which they are positioned is not a coincidence. That's because it represents the flow of activity in the business. It illustrates perfectly the journey of a patient and how every one of those four departments have a role to play in ensuring that the patient completes the journey with you.

Here's how it all comes together:

MARKETING STARTS THE PLAY

It is the job of the **marketing** team to spark the initial interest and awareness that your service or clinic even exists. Not much can happen if people do not know you exist, and yet most physical therapy clinics sadly try to operate without a marketing dept.

The skillsets required of the marketing person include copywriting, strategy, and tactical know-how of things like Facebook and Google. Then there are the more emotional skills required, those such as empathy and the understanding of emotional and psychological triggers of your target market - those people you've identified. The marketing people are given the responsibility of getting the right message out to the right people by using the right platform in the most economical way.

Marketing done right (as I explain in the *"New Patient Accelerator Method Book"*, www.paulsmarketingbook.com) is about generating interest from people with problems you can solve. It's about getting leads. It is not about selling appointments or asking people to call and book sessions.

No, if marketing is doing a good job, the phone will start to ring with people making inquires. Marketing is about getting people to raise their hand, indicating an interest in wanting to know more about how you can help them to solve their problems.

MARKETING PASSES TO SALES

This is where the **sales** people/dept. step in. If the phone rings with inquires, someone has to have the skills to be able to communicate and talk to that person in a way that makes it more likely they will want to take the next step with you – become a paying patient.

The sales person is continuing the conversation started by the marketing department; they are confirming that the outcome promised in the marketing can be delivered. Essentially, the sales people are talking to those folks who see an ad in the newspaper, who show an interest at a local event, or who see you on Facebook. They are asking value driven questions, responding to objections over cost, confirming suitability for physical therapy, and ultimately helping people make good decisions that lead them to booking appointments with you.

So, marketing starts the play. And to use a football analogy, marketing then passes the ball to the sales people to make the next move. The people in the sales dept. have very different skills and personalities, and therefore could never be expected to do both jobs (long term). Good sales people need to be able to handle rejection, display empathy, communicate value, and be relentless in their pursuit of an outcome – amongst many others.

I often refer to my sales dept. as the **Nurture or Follow Up** team, because that is ultimately what they do; they follow up on inquires. They make more revenue likely because they are there to help prospects move from inquiry to paying patient, however long it takes. One of my favorite sayings is "the fortune is in the follow up".

That's because people often need more than one conversation before saying yes to you. You've got to have someone in your clinic having this dialogue for you or you're losing a small fortune.

Last thing on this: do not get confused with what a sales dept. is. It is simply one or two people in your office who are able to talk confidently to patients who are, at first, a little tentative and skeptical about paying for your services. Whoever it is that is hired to do this role for you must be skilled enough to be able to talk to these people, and, importantly, in a way that increases the likelihood of an appointment being made.

PAUL'S BOLD STATEMENT ABOUT THE FUTURE OF THE PROFESSION

As the profession crosses the frontier from relying on referrals from doctors and low copays to direct marketing and cash pay or higher copays, it is now vital to have this type of role, (Nurture/Follow up role), filled by the right person in your office. The objections are coming more frequently; the resistance to treatment plans and the resentment to higher costs are already a problem. This means a different type of person is required, not necessarily the pleasant guy or girl you'd typically employ to sit at the front desk – you need someone with very different skills.

I am going to go on record and tell you that from the hundreds of clinics I have worked with, <u>this *is* the problem that needs solving for most of them to be able to grow.</u>

Do not confuse being nice, polite, and efficient, with being able to hold a real conversation about money, the cost of physical therapy, and the benefits of paying for it.

Do not confuse this role with a "client care coordinator" or anything like that – this is a specific role for someone with specific skills in selling.

What is more, realize that if people say "no", if the right person is hired, it is possible to get them to say "yes!" It is only when someone says "yes" that you get to actually make any money. That is why you need someone who is good at it. Clinical skills are no match for an objection over cost from a discouraged patient who is living life pay-cheque to pay-cheque, i.e. most of the world.

In the years after this book is published, I am 100% certain that costs will not be going down. That is why I am confident about saying that getting this department filled with the right person is likely to be the no.1 reason your clinic prospers or struggles and eventually dies.

For that reason alone, it could be the no.1 reason you'll be glad you picked up this book.

SALES PASSES TO OPERATIONS TO FULFILL

With the sales/nurture people doing their job, interested prospects are now committed and happy to arrive at their first appointment. And so it's over to the **operations** department to fulfill on the promise made by the sales person.

This is where the "traditional" front of house person starts to talk to them about suitable appointments, how to get to the clinic, where to park, explains how billing works, and so on. With that taken care of, the other half of the operations department now steps up – the physical therapist.

So far, the process is efficient and the patient is happy. The marketing sparked an interest, the sales person confirmed suitability, and the front of house explained all of the requirements and started to create the experience the patient is looking forward to receiving.

Everything is working well to this point. It's now over to the physical therapist who has just one job to do, and that can be summed up in five words:

"Do not screw it up!"

Think about it… the patient is in your world now. Everyone has done their job well so far. It is now up to the physical therapist to do the easiest job in the world: get the patient the outcome that the physical therapist has trained for years at school to be able to do!

Ease the pain, get the movement back, help them walk further with less pain, sleep longer, get off pills, avoid surgery – whatever it is that they want to do (that was promised in the marketing), just give it to them! Apply your skills and get the result the patient wants.

Their only job is to get results that keep patients happy and coming back. It is the easiest job, by far. How can I say this? Because of all of the struggles that business owners tell me they are going through, I've never had a single one tell me that the reason they're not making a profit is because they couldn't get patients better.

"I am not a very good clinician and that is why my business is struggling" are words I have never heard. Ever.

It is more often than not the complete opposite:

"When they hear about me – they never want to leave."

Or, *"If I could just get more patients, everything would be great!"*

This is suggestive of a marketing problem. To be precise, it's usually a lack of marketing problem. And that emphasizes my point; the therapist's job is to keep the patients. And on the whole, most do it well. They do it even better if they're backed by a great marketing message, a strong sales person, and a great front of house person with the time to put people at ease when they arrive in your clinic.

I tell my physical therapists regularly that they have no idea how lucky they are working at my clinics; not because it is "me" they are working for, but because they have a marketing department that finds our perfect patients; they have a sales person (two in fact!) who answer all of the objections in advance of the first session, thereby turning skeptics into easy-to-work-with patients.

What's more, they have an amazing front of house team whose job it is to "WOW" people from the moment they walk through the door. They do it that well that people will often express their sorrow for leaving once their treatment ends. All of this combined means it's harder for the therapist to fail than it is to succeed.

OPERATIONS PASSES THE BALL TO FINANCE

Next up, the ball is passed to **finance**; if marketing has sparked the interest, sales has converted that initial interest to commitment and the physical therapist has done what we promised, it's now time for you to get paid. This is where the people in finance (or accounts/billing as some would call it) step into the play.

The people in finance will do the necessities such as bill insurance, create invoices or super bills, etc. That means you're going to get paid, and hopefully at 20-25% more than what it costs to do all of that which we have just described above. I.e. you're going to make a nice healthy profit and see a return on your assets (staff).

YOU DO NOT NEED TO START WITH ALL THE SEATS FILLED WITH THE PERFECT PERSON

Finally, as you look at that organizational structure, I am aware that it is tempting to get overwhelmed or think that you should have all of the positions filled right away. You don't. If you're new in business, let this be the map that guides your future hiring choices.

The ideal situation is that you have someone appropriately skilled in each of those positions. But, "ideal" is not always available for a small business owner like you and I. You'll fill them as the need becomes obvious, demand increases, or you've made a strategic decision to scale quickly.

Know this: getting the right people in the right seats is possibly your most important job as a business owner, but I can tell you from experience that it is not how you'll get started. In the beginning it's ok to have your front desk person helping you out with marketing, doing follow up calls, and chasing up invoices for you.

You can start there, but you can't stay there.

If you're new in business, please don't overlook this lesson I am sharing. And if you're an experienced business owner, in business for more than five years, I bet that the guy or girl at your front desk right now is most likely doing all of these different things for you.

If so, now you know why you're stuck. Now you know why the person in that role keeps quitting. Now you know why you can never seem to get past an invisible ceiling in your business. You are asking a quarterback to play every role on the field – on the same day!

Seriously, for most established clinics, what they need more than anything is to take a closer look at who they have and in what seats they are they sitting. If you are expecting Sally at your front desk to provide an exceptional customer experience, to be able to answer objections about money, balance your books, chase un-paid bills, AND do your clinics marketing for you – then that's why you're stuck!

All of those tasks require completely different skill sets, and it's no wonder that Sally looks stressed and tired, and that you've had to replace her four times in two years. It's not her – it's that what you are asking her to do is simply not sustainable. What is more, her great personality does not appear to be brought to work as much as it used to.

So, there you have it. That's how every successful company is structured. That is how all successful companies and their departments are interconnected. Something to think over as you decide on who is going to be your next hire and when, which, coincidentally is the topic of the next chapter.

Come with me and we'll talk more specifically about all of the **different roles** required in a successful physical therapy clinic, and moreover, what they should each do…

4

WHO TO HIRE AND WHEN

Now that you know how your company should be structured, let's look more specifically at who you should hire (the types of roles you will need to be filling), and when you should hire (in what order).

Broadly speaking, there are really only six roles that you'll need to fill at your practice. The ones I will discuss are likely to be sufficient for 99% of the people reading this book, 99% of the time. That's because there's really only a finite number of positions that need filling in any company. Everything else is likely to be same position, just with an elaborate title that the boss chose to make a role seem more appealing or appease the staff. The problem is, however, it often confuses everyone else.

There's a great saying that I love: "if you want to multiply, simplify". It's relevant here, because although getting creative with job titles can be gratifying, all this does in a growing company is waste time and energy that could be better spent elsewhere.

I once had a very mild and light-hearted disagreement with a staff member in my marketing company on this exact topic. We produce a monthly marketing newsletter (titled, *Cash is King*), and in the newsletter I positioned her as "Community Manageress." Why? Because she manages the community of readers from all over the world.

I agree, it wasn't the most creative title I could have come up with, but to consider anything else would have taken me too long to think about. As the story goes, she didn't like the title. She said "it didn't suit her". She asked if she could change it and I told her she could call herself anything she wants. I don't really care what title she carries. I only care what she does. The rest is irrelevant to me, and, in fact, a complete waste of my energy to get involved in or to have to think about.

Believe me, if you're at the helm of growing a company, there are many more things you should be concerning yourself with other than titles of roles. With that said, I won't be getting too imaginative with the names of the roles I'll be describing in this chapter. If I use the words "physical therapist" or "front desk person" (and so on), I think you'll know what I mean…

SIX SPECIFIC ROLES THAT YOU NEED TO FILL

So, let's look more specifically at the roles/positions that you need to fill at your clinic. Then, after that, I'll show you what the company organizational chart at my clinic (the *Paul Gough Physio Rooms*) currently looks like, and you can see how these 6 different roles are visualized in a clinic. What is more I'll answer the question of **who** you hire first, at the end of this chapter.

1. PHYSICAL THERAPIST (OPERATIONS)

Your therapists sit in the operations department. Their primary job is to ensure that the patient gets the outcome promised to them by your sales and marketing team i.e. being able to walk further with less pain.

As I've mentioned a few times in the book already, it is very common to think that the physical therapist should be in charge of filling up their own case-load. I think that is madness. I've seen many clinic owners insist on their clinicians being responsible for their own case-load – and later live to regret. You give them the confidence and force them to figure out how-to acquire their own patients, and it won't be long before they leave with all their patients and set up down the street in competition against you. Why wouldn't the physical therapist do it? All that stands in the way of most opening their own clinic – is their own case load and knowing how to keep it topped up.

To stop that from happening, the answer is to create a marketing system that delivers patients independent of who the physical therapist is. Don't stop them from doing things like community events or talks on your behalf – but do not ask them to set it all do. Do not ask them to create the system to make the event happen. They can fulfill it, but you establish it. That means anyone in the future who you hire can step in and fulfill such an event if an when your therapists leave.

Here's my best tip: hire physical therapists solely to do what they want to do: treat patients. You create a marketing system to keep them busy. If they leave you, you have still got the marketing system and as a result, you'll be able to easily fill up the next therapist.

2. FRONT OF HOUSE/ADMIN (OPERATIONS)

This is your traditional guy or girl who sits at your front desk. They are in operations and work in tandem with the physical therapist to ensure that the patient gets an outcome they're happy to pay for. This is the role that is, in my humble opinion, perhaps <u>the most important.</u> It's the one that the physical therapists often take for granted (until a good one arrives).

This person has the computer in front of them, files all around, the phone on their desk, and they're usually expected to do everything from:

- Meeting and greeting new patients – as well as making tea and coffee

- Billing and sending out bills

- Answering the phone and putting the one person on hold while booking an appointment for a patient who has just finished their session

- Confirming appointments and ringing drop offs

- Ensuring that schedules are utilized correctly

- Following up on leads

- Returning faxes to doctors and talking to insurance companies for authorization

- Sending emails with directions to patients and even, possibly, doing the clinics social media and doing a bit of marketing…

…and anything else that the owner can throw at them.

This is one of, if not the most, pivotal roles in the clinic, and yet the person doing it is hardly ever allowed the opportunity to be successful at it – simply because they're expected to do too much. They often don't really know what their job even is.

They are not given the best chance to be successful because they don't ever know what it is they should be prioritizing. As a result, a little bit of everything gets done with very little success. At my clinic, this role has one key objective, and that is to provide a WOW factor experience to every patient they come into contact with. I want them to give all patients an incredible customer experience. Whether it is on the phone, via an email, SMS, or when the patient arrives for an appointment, all of their attention must go to this person. Everything else must stop. It is this person's job to spend

20-30 minutes on the first phone call with a patient, ensuring they're happy and understand the process.

Likewise, when the patients arrive at the clinic I, want the front desk person free to be able to engage and connect with them; to get to know people over and above just being patients. They're sending personal SMS/TEXT reminders (<u>not</u> automated), and, if the situation requires it, they're even allowed to leave their desk and sit next to the patient and enjoy a cup of coffee and have a chat with the patient while they wait for their appointment.

Anything else that they get done is a bonus. The patient and how they are made to feel is the No.1 priority, and as a result we are staffed (and priced) appropriately.

If you are reading this and thinking, *"I'd love to do this, but we don't have the staff"*, then it's simple – hire.

And if your next excuse is *"but I can't afford to"*, then it's simple; raise your fees.

And if you're next excuse is, *"but I can't, I'm paid by insurance"*, it's simple – drop the worst payers and start charging cash so that you can <u>provide the type of service that people want to pay for</u>.

At my clinic, the front of house person deals exclusively with what I call "inbound" phone calls. That is, people calling to book appointments who already know, like, and trust us, or patients who want to re-arrange appointments. The front of house/admin people are not calling the leads/inquires that come in from the clinics direct marketing. That is done by the people in the next role:

3. FOLLOW UP/LEAD NURTURE (SALES)

This person sits in the sales department, as seen on the organizational chart. Their job is to talk to all of the leads/prospective inquires that come from the direct to public marketing campaigns we run on Google, Facebook, in the newspapers and so on.

Now, if you are reading this and you are not sure what a lead/prospect is, then I strongly suggest you read (or re-read) my marketing book, namely *"New Patient Accelerator Method"* (**www.PaulsMarketingBook.com**) It'll help you understand the different types of patients and how you can have them calling you. More specifically, it will help you understand where the patient is on their buying journey.

For example, when a new patient is calling you at 9.05am tomorrow morning, they want to (or are close to) booking an appointment. It's called inbound because that person is calling "into" your clinic. These people are usually easy to talk to; they've actively looked for you and have willingly made the decision to call you. They're likely already bought into you and your message, therefore the person at the front desk can handle it. There's usually not that much selling or that many challenging objections to be dealt with when speaking to this type of patient.

At first, you can get going and even survive on people calling you inbound via word of mouth, doctors, good will, etc. But in the end, if you continue to rely on this type of patient, you will get *stuck*. There are simply not enough patients out there who know what we do will confidently call up and be ready to book.

That makes it difficult to grow or scale, and so you have to move towards marketing directly to public who may not know, like or trust you. These are the people in Group 2 (that I described in my *Accelerator* book); they are out there and living with problems you can help with, but they just do not consider you as an option, yet. However, if you do your marketing right you'll gain their interest.

These people need nurturing, and their inquiries often need to be followed up on more than once (hence why I call it the Follow

Up or Nurture role). With the right person talking to them on the phone, you'll soon get the appointments.

As I said earlier, this person in the sales department is the vital missing link in most clinics. It's sad, but true that most people running clinics never even consider this person to be needed – and that is because they're never doing any real marketing. Most clinics are waiting all day for the phone to ring, only for it to be answered by the guy or girl at the front desk. And yet, it never rings as frequently as the owner would like.

What is more, most owners never stop to consider that "no" doesn't actually mean "no". It just means "no, not right now".

It means "no" because, right now, "I don't know enough or feel confident enough to say yes". But, if you spend some time with them and help them feel more confident enough to say "yes", then guess what? ... "No" *does* become "yes".

For most businesses reading this, and depending upon your level of inquiries, having this person will become the critical missing link that can likely add $100,000's to your bottom line. And that is no exaggeration.

This role is 100% about talking to leads who make inquiries - those folks who are skeptical, who tentatively download a free report on Facebook, or fill out a form on your website late at night. They are building relationships with people who may not currently see the value, who may have some price concerns or questions that they need addressed, for example, before they will invest the type of money that you charge.

Basically, most all of the people in your town.

If you take nothing else from this book, it should be the realization that if you are getting push-back, patients don't seem to want to pay, or don't see your value, won't commit, or keep going elsewhere because it's "cheaper", then this nurture person will solve that problem for you.

What is funny is when I point this out to the clinic owners who buy my courses or programs; nearly all of them took more than one email, one podcast or one webinar to get comfortable with me and confident enough to buy something like my New Patient Accelerator program or join my Cash Club program. As I candidly point out to each of them, why is it any different for your patients? What makes it ok for them to need the time to get comfortable with buying something – but it not be ok for the same process to happen with their patients?

Of course, there is no difference. And it's only when it is pointed out that we – even as confident business owners – rarely make impulsive decisions to buy things does the penny drop that this is something to consider for their own clinic. Something that is an absolute pre-requisite if you really want to help more people while simultaneously making your clinic more profitable.

Hint: next time you make an inquiry with a company and they call you back in two days' time if you didn't buy from them (if not sooner), that's the follow up person going to work on your inquiry. Why not put one to work for you?

4. MARKETING ASSISTANT

Next up is the marketing person; trying to grow any business without someone in there who can market the business is like buying a car thinking you can drive it without putting any gas in it. It is like building a $10,000,000 shopping mall and putting it in the middle of nowhere, then expecting people to find it. It is crazy. And yet so many do it.

This person's job is to craft the appropriate marketing message, one that will resonate with the clinic's perfect patient. They have to ensure an appropriate number of new leads and inquires arrive each week (over and above word of mouth).

<u>Without</u> new leads and inquires coming in, your clinic is stuck. There's then no need for a follow up or sales person, and you're back to relying upon the slow, old fashioned methods of word of mouth or past patients coming back. If you don't get the people through the doors there's no one for the operational team to service.

No operations, no finance. No finance, no cheques to cash. No cheques to cash, no business.

This is a very important role, and if you're just starting out, here's my tip on where to find this person today:

Look in the <u>mirror</u> – they are staring right back at you.

That's right. At first, the marketing assistant needs to be you. You must become the marketer of the business. The best advice I can give anyone in business is to start thinking of themselves as a marketer of their business. The most successful companies I have studied all have one thing in common: the founder is a brilliant marketer. Whether it was Steve Jobs at Apple or Walt at Disney, they were over and above all other things, world class at marketing.

Marketing is a skill that can be learned, just like dry needling or massage. Take the courses and classes, read the books, go to the seminars, and when you understand how to market your clinic correctly, then and only then is the time to bring in someone to help you.

The absolute worst thing you can do is hire someone who has a "marketing degree" or give the responsibility to someone who "knows social media", or, just as bad, outsource it to a big ad agency who have absolutely no clue how to market to attract patients that will want to pay. That is called abdication. Business owners must never abdicate. You must first master the strategy and then, once you understand it, outsource the tactics.

5. FINANCE (DIFFERENT FROM BILLING)

As you grow, particularly as you start to scale, you'll want to consider people helping you with billing and managing your cash flow.

Start with a bookkeeper that will do tasks like send out invoices, chase payments, and even keep Quick Books/Sage up to date for you. This is a $15/20 per hour role, so do not do it yourself for too long (and don't expect your front desk to do it all either). Then, as you grow, and the cash activities (and risk) in your business escalate, bring in someone with more skills who will protect you as you grow.

At my clinic, when we hit $1m in annual revenue I brought in a full-time finance person who sat above (in the org chart) the part time booker keeper/billing person that I already had. This person does so much more for me than just billing and chasing down owed money; he is involved in preparing my weekly, monthly, quarterly, and yearly management reports.

These are very different from reports prepared for accountants/tax purposes, and they are very different from those obtained inside Quick Books or Sage. They include profit and loss statements, monthly balance sheets, updating the budget and variance analysis, the statements of cash, accounts receivable days, and preparing a rolling 13-week cash flow forecast - so that we don't run out of cash when we want to invest or grow. He is a liaison with my tax attorneys (in the UK and USA), and keeps me updated with all things financial in the clinic.

This has been one of the greatest hires I've ever made.

I've got so much more information at my disposal about how my clinics are doing, and this is one of the reasons I'm able to keep my clinics growing in the UK while residing in the USA for most of the year.

I have my entire business activity condensed into a spreadsheet that I can read from anywhere in the world, thereafter making the decisions that are required of me.

This person is talking to the bookkeeper, keeping an eye on expenses, and always ensuring that we're never going over the budget on any of the expense line items that I've set. Crucially, this person ensures that there's money in the bank to meet payroll. It may take a few years to get to this point – but it once you do, it's worth investing in.

6. OPERATIONS MANAGER/GENERAL MANAGER/ CLINIC DIRECTOR

At my clinic, because I am not "in the business" anymore day to day (even though I still own it and make decisions), I chose to hire a General/Operations Manager. This is a non-clinical person who is managing my business for me. I know it is common practice to appoint a leading physical therapist as the clinic director, but for all sorts of reasons, I do not think it is the best strategy.

First of all, just because they are the best physical therapist does not mean that they can do all of the things required of a General Manager. These things include managing people, tracking KPI's, hiring and firing, being meticulous with processes, being attentive to detail, and being able to "police" over the clinic in the owner's absence (which is <u>just some</u> of what is required by a GM).

Secondly, they would be the highest paid Operations/General Manager – ever. And that would make their position very inefficient.

The cost of hiring a good manger, with proven experience of being able to plan, manage people, track and understand KPI's, etc., would be significantly less than having someone who is a qualified physical therapist do it for you (and they'd most likely do it better).

Great soccer players rarely become good managers. Great nurses rarely make great managers of the ward. Great sales people rarely become great managers of sales people. That is because the skills required to do these roles are wildly different.

As I see so many clinic owners trying to exit the day to day running of their business and leave it to a clinic director, the primary reason they can't get fully away from the business is because of the clinic director; they've hired someone with the wrong skills and not set clear expectations of what is required.

Why does it happen so much in physical therapy? Well, usually it's because of the "it's always been done this way" mentality which is rarely a good reason to do anything. And secondly, there's little if any understanding of the outcomes required of someone in that position to allow the owner to ever be freed up. There's a failure to consider the tasks and skills required of someone in that position and as a result they are always pulled back in to fight another fire that the clinic director couldn't deal with. This is something we will come on to in chapter 7.

Truth be told, at my clinic I promoted a lady to the General Managers role quite reluctantly. Not because I didn't want to give her the role, but because I was worried I was promoting her out of the role she was already great at.

I spent a year or so thinking over whether it was the right decision for her to be hired for this new position. It was only after I looked critically at all of the things she would be required to do in the role, and then asked myself daily if she had somewhere in the past demonstrated to me that she could do all of those roles excellently, that things became clearer. In the end, I believed that she could, and hence why I took her off the front desk and moved her into a management role. She's been a revelation ever since.

The point is this: I didn't do it 'just because' I thought she was the best front desk person, or because she had been with me the longest. I did it because I knew what the role required (outcomes) and saw proof of her being able to achieve the tasks required of the role.

That is the big difference from appointing my best physical therapist as manager just because she's got the best diagnostic skills or most experience – even best personality. Of course, however, I do have a head physical therapist who all of the other clinicians can go to and ask questions of. He sits at the top of the org chart, on the clinical side of the Operations Department.

Here's how it works: if there are any issues in the clinical team (physical therapists, sports therapist, and massage therapist), they'll report to the head of clinical, who will report it to the General Manager, who will, if needs be, report it to me.

There's a chain of command - everyone knows their roles, who to talk to, and when. I rarely ever speak to anyone but the people in the head of the four major departments. Of course, I say hello to everyone when I am in the clinic, but if it is an issue with the clinic, or I am talking about developing it, I am going to the heads of operations, finance, marketing and sales first. It is their job to pass the message to the appropriate person below them in the org chart.

With the right company structure (as outlined in chapter 3), it makes it very easy to own a business that runs without your day-to-day involvement.

CLARIFYING WHO IS SELLING – AND WHEN

Before I move on, I just want to make something clear: when I say that physical therapists and front desk "shouldn't be selling", I do not mean it literally. Every single person in your organization is constantly selling. Selling your value, your message, and what makes you different.

There's not a single person in life that isn't, or shouldn't, constantly be selling. Even if it's selling yourself to the girl or guy of your dreams, that someone who you eventually want to marry –

and then stay married to – you are still selling your qualities over another option he or she might have.

Another example: my 5-year-old son Harry is constantly selling to me. He is selling me on getting him a TV in his room, getting a dog, wanting an ice cream cone, or to do stuff that he knows I might say no to first time round. Have you noticed how kids don't just ask you for stuff and then take no for the answer?

No, they really sell why they want it, and they are good at helping you see why they should get it. And moreover, they do it more than once, even after you've said no ten times. They have a great way of *nurturing* you to the point that you want to say yes, despite saying no to start with. The "fortune is in the follow up", everywhere in life.

Here's the point: doing this doesn't mean that when you meet the guy or the girl of your dreams you were a "salesperson". Or, when Harry is putting his case forward as to why I should let him have a dog, that he is a professional sales person. Far from it. That is just what he has to do to get what he wants in life.

It is the same with all of your staff. Even my finance guy who sits in the back office regularly walks through the clinic and comes into contact with my patients. He has to act and talk in a way that presents the clinic in a positive light. If he doesn't, it could cause patients to drop off or not come back because of how he made them feel.

The bottom line is that yes, in an evaluation, on the phone, when presenting a plan of care, your staff are selling or marketing for you. But they're not in the same kind of situation as the person in the sales or marketing dept. whose job it is to think up incredibly powerful headlines for newspaper ads, or handle money objections, or skepticism about the value of physical therapy.

Please do not confuse this. You are putting people with the right skills in the appropriate seats. However, you and everyone in your clinic are always selling your value just like every human on earth is always selling his or hers. Always and forever. The day that you stop is the day you'll go out of business.

HOW I STRUCTURE MY OWN CLINIC

At the beginning of the chapter I promised you a look at how my company org chart looks. Well, here it is. The image below shows you how the Paul Gough Physio Room is structured:

FIG.6 PAUL GOUGH PHYSIO ROOMS ORG CHART

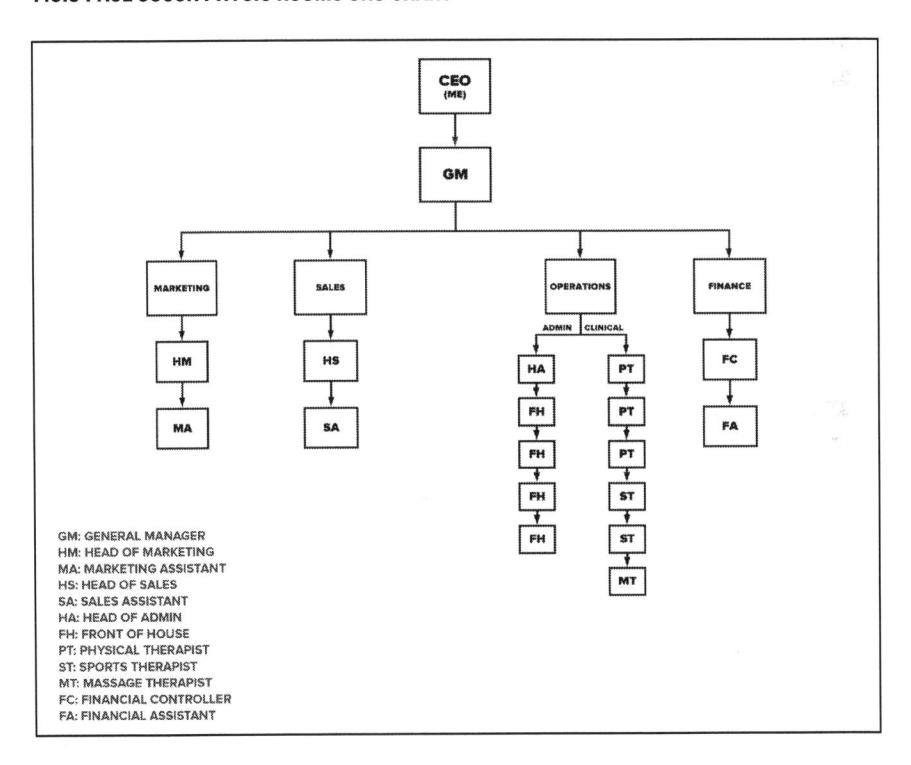

```
                        CEO
                        (ME)
                         |
                         GM
    _____|_____
    |           |              |              |
MARKETING     SALES       OPERATIONS       FINANCE
    |           |         ADMIN|CLINICAL       |
    HM          HS         HA     PT           FC
    |           |          |      |            |
    MA          SA         FH     PT           FA
                           |      |
                           FH     PT
                           |      |
                           FH     ST
                           |      |
                           FH     ST
                                  |
                                  MT
```

GM: GENERAL MANAGER
HM: HEAD OF MARKETING
MA: MARKETING ASSISTANT
HS: HEAD OF SALES
SA: SALES ASSISTANT
HA: HEAD OF ADMIN
FH: FRONT OF HOUSE
PT: PHYSICAL THERAPIST
ST: SPORTS THERAPIST
MT: MASSAGE THERAPIST
FC: FINANCIAL CONTROLLER
FA: FINANCIAL ASSISTANT

As you can see, I've got all four major departments across the top filled. I won't use their names as it'll get confusing and I don't want to have to keep reprinting this book - you never know when one may need to be moved out and I'll need to follow this system again myself...

In addition to the four major departments, you'll notice that I have a General Manager (GM) who sits in between me and those major departments. This is the person that I speak to most. This person's role as GM is to communicate with everyone below her.

She's talking to the person in marketing, talking to her assistant in sales about how the conversions and upsells are going (sales), and talking to the finance guy about things like cash flow and asking if we've got money in the account for payroll. She's talking to the Head PT and Head of Admin to ensure that things like schedules are utilized correctly, that the patients are showing up, and that cancels or no-shows are above the level we set.

As you look below the top line, you'll see there's a long list of physical therapists, sports therapists, and massage therapists running down underneath the operations department. All of those people on the right-hand side of operations are in clinical. If any of those people have an issue, need to speak to someone, or have a concern, then it is the guy at the top they talk to. Displayed in the org chart as Head PT (HP).

On the left-hand side of operations is the Head of Admin. This person is displayed as HA, and if anyone in that department has any issues like sickness, wants vacations, wants something clarified, or wants to share something, they'll do it with HA. It is then the job of HA to share it with the GM, who, if she deems necessary, shares it with the CEO (me) during our weekly meeting.

And that's it. That is how simple, but stunningly effective my company structure is.

Everyone is hired for the right role, one that they are skilled enough to perform. They're all given quantifiable standards (measurable outcomes) to hit, and they're monitored appropriately as to how they are doing (accountability). The people in operations are delivering on the promise made by marketing and sales people. If anyone feels unable to do their job or are not happy, they talk to the person above them, who talks to the person above them. From there it gets dealt with, or it gets escalated to me.

At the time of writing, I've run my business for over 5 years now without having a phone line in my personal office. I rarely, if ever, respond to any emails from anyone in the clinic. They all know not to waste their time, as I won't respond for days. Since the day I started to hire correctly, monitor their work by ensuring KPI's, and critical driver standards (all to be discussed) were put in place, I've had a six-figure profitable business year on year – and without having to be there every day.

I am rarely, if ever, putting out fires. And if one starts, I can see the person with the match and deal with it appropriately. When I tell you that there is another to way to run a business, one that doesn't involve the chaos and madness that most clinic owners are engulfed in daily, <u>I mean it.</u> It requires the right people hired into the right company structure – hired in the right order by a leader – that's you – prepared to call it tight and hold them accountable.

WHO TO HIRE FIRST?

So, who should you hire first? What should the order be? Is it a physical therapist or a front desk person?

That is a common question I get asked, and there are a lot of opinions on this, but there's only one answer... and that's to hire a front of house person.

Think about it: if you keep hiring physical therapists, who is going to answer the phone and deal with all of the extra work that comes with more patients? You? Are you going to stop doing $200 per hour work and start doing $15 per hour work? Why would anyone do that?

What is more, anyone who does this is making the mistake of thinking that front of house/admin are not revenue generators. Your accountant will tell you that they're not, but I can tell you they are.

(As I said in Chapter 2, <u>never</u> ask an accountant for advice on growing your company).

If you keep adding therapists then, yes, in the beginning they will make more revenue. However, it will come at the price of creating a real business that has a strong foundation that you can grow from.

Choosing a therapist over an admin feels easier, as it assumes that you're not going to be out of pocket. But it's a short-term fix. Bringing in an admin to meet and greet patients is the beginning of something that is bigger than just you; something bigger than just providing physical therapy. It is the start of you creating better experiences for patients.

And it is only when you move into the business of providing better "experiences" for people that business growth becomes easier. If it is all about physical therapy then you'll remain a commodity. You'll always feel like you're being price shopped or have difficulty raising your rates.

I've said it many times publicly: any clinic owner who thinks that patients are only coming to get physical therapy because they're a great clinician, needs to get a reality check. Business is about people. All commerce is about people doing business with people. It's not just about having problems solved – it's about <u>how</u> the problem is solved. The people are the how.

Rushing people in and out for their treatment is a transaction. Having the time allocated to really get to know people makes them feel special – that is what they remember. That is why they come back. That is why they tell more people about you. The key word is time. That's the thing that humans value more than anything, and when you give it to someone they can really feel it. Bring the right person onto your front desk and you'll achieve this. What is more, you've just given your patients another reason to come and see you; and that reason is the person at the front desk who is building their own relationship with your patients. The more relationships they have in your clinic the harder it is for them not to want to come back. That is where the profit is for you.

Given the right time and in the right company structure, your front of house person is able to spend time with patients and in doing so, is finding out very different things about those patients than they'll ever tell you or their therapist. If you've never experienced people wanting to book appointments with you *just* for an excuse to spend time with your front desk person, then you've got the wrong front desk people.

You might have the right person to send emails and be efficient – but, you've definitely not got a revenue generator in that seat. The right person on your front desk pays for themselves many times over. At my clinic the total bill is $250; this is made up of $150 to see the physical therapist and an additional $100 for the great experience we provide and the people you'll meet. I assure you, if you give it to them, people are happy to pay more for the right experience.

If your patients aren't happy to pay higher than normal fees then it's another sign/symptom that you're missing something; you're probably lacking the right experience they want to pay for.

For all those reasons and more, it is my humble opinion that hiring a great front desk person first is the best option.

With the "big picture" stuff covered, let's get on with the recruitment and hiring process. "Vision without action is just a dream", and, "action without a plan is a nightmare". That is why your hiring process must start with a detailed plan.

It is the first step (of six) in the Outcomes Based Hiring Model we're going to work through together to help you find world-class staff that you can trust. Turn over to the next page to see all six of the steps - and then we'll move to the next page thereafter to start creating that plan…

THE OUTCOMES BASED HIRING SYSTEM FOR PHYSICAL THERAPY CLINICS

STEP 1:
CREATE THE HIRING PLAN

STEP 2:
ESTABLISH THE FINANCIAL METRIC OF SUCCESS

STEP 3:
CREATE THE SUCCESS DESCRIPTION
(OUTCOMES, TASKS, MEASURE, SKILLS)

STEP 4:
CREATE THE JOB AD
(AND WHERE TO POST IT)

STEP 5:
THE 6-PART INTERVIEW PROCESS
(AND WHAT QUESTIONS TO ASK)

STEP 6:
THE 7, 30, AND 90-DAY ONBOARDING PROCESS

Ok, there's the six steps in this process - now turn to the next page and I'll teach you how to do it...

5

STEP 1/6: HOW TO CREATE YOUR HIRING PLAN

"Occam's Razor" is a theory that suggests when faced with two different ways to achieve the same outcome, you should always choose the simplest. The simplest way to lose weight is to just *put down the fork*, and the simplest way to improve your hiring success is to spend more time thinking about it. Simply take more time to create a detailed plan that you'll follow - and watch your hiring success odds increase.

Doing that involves considering things like what you are hiring for, who it is that you really want, when you will need those people, and how much you need to spend. Then, knowing all of that, create a job ad that narrows down the candidate pool exclusively to those capable of doing the job as you need.

That is the plan that we're about to create in this chapter

But please don't be fooled by how simplistic it sounds. It is simple, but there's a big difference between common sense and common practice, and that's why I am inserting "create the hiring plan" right at the start of the process. Do not be tempted to skip this part, as it will cost you dearly later on.

Now, when making a hiring plan there are three things to consider:

1. Time
2. Money
3. Compensation

Let's look at each one more closely:

CONSIDERATION #1: TIME

If you think about how most people hire, they wait until they really need someone. They leave it until the business need is pressing. But, that's the problem. It's easy to get caught up in a vicious cycle of doing all of the stuff you need your new hire to do, and because of that you're too busy to find the time to actually go out and hire them (to do all of the stuff you currently are).

This often goes on for weeks, and it is only when the frustration reaches boiling point that the owner decides it's time to do something and hire someone. At this point, anyone will do, and so one of the most common hiring mistakes is made.

The way to avoid being trapped like this is to plan <u>annually</u>.

Business planning is something that is grossly underestimated and often ignored. The reason being because it doesn't feel like much is achieved when you sit and plan. Yet, anyone who actually does it knows that the value of planning comes weeks and months later when your business is running smoothly – and according to plan.

Only people who have *never* had a plan for their business would tell you that they're too busy to plan; those who *are* annual planners will tell you that they're never too busy to plan – and this is precisely *because* they plan.

The best hiring situation to be in is when you are in preparation for more success, not when you are already successful and the phone is ringing off the hook. I call this planning for success. Most people plan for nothing; they wish for better or hope for more, but usually get much the same as what they got last year - the same as the year before and the year before that.

Here's how I do it: at the end of every year I sit down on my own for two days and plan for success. I dedicate that time to creating a budget for my business. A budget is simply a set of assumptions about what I expect to achieve financially. It is what I want to happen. I put down on paper a figure, and alongside that figure I work out what has to happen to make it happen. As in, what activity has to take place and who has to be responsible for it.

A great plan without the right resources is doomed to fail. That is why I must consider what the additional marketing activities need to be (if I want to grow) and what stress all of that would add to the business. Then I can think about staff; are we staffed appropriately to handle the marketing and sales activities that would be required to hit the goal?

If my answer is that we would not be able to cope with the increased demand of phone calls and inquires (from the marketing activities I have planned), then, as part of my annual plan, I am also writing down when I will need to start the hiring process to be ready for the increase.

Doing this means that I am never hiring on impulse. I have an idea of when I will need to be hiring and so the hiring process does not spook me. It is all planned months ahead of time.

Now, of course, it doesn't always transpire that I get my assumptions right every time. But the fact that I sit down and do it means that I am going to get it right more often than not. And, I am actually ready for it when it happens.

What you will learn from me as you move through this book (and any of my previous or future books in this series), is that success in business is actually not that difficult. The hardest part is not necessarily all of the things that people worry about, such as marketing, hiring, or cash flow, but having the discipline to sit down and think and plan.

Realistically, how many people do that? Very few, is my bet. And how many businesses struggle? The answer is, "a lot". The correlation between the two should not be overlooked.

Side note: at the time of writing this book I am simultaneously in the process of creating a new 2-day in-person workshop dedicated to creating a Business Plan. Specifically, "How to Create a Business Plan to Prepare For Growth" – if you are interested in attending, send an email to paul@paulgough.com and we'll get the dates and more information to you.

Now truth be told, I am not very good at this planning and thinking thing. Entrepreneurs do find it difficult. It means I find it a struggle to do it, but I do it anyway because I know my business is better as a result of the planning that I do.

More than anything really, I want to be creating a new marketing campaign or thinking up something new to sell. I enjoy those things, but they are not always the best use of my time. Sitting down and taking the time to do things like think and plan for the 12 months ahead, is difficult. It is not sexy; it is not instantly gratifying, but it is very profitable and saves you from getting into bad situations that cost you more time and more money for not doing so.

This is a discipline that I have had to force myself to become better at, and it is something that I'll have to work at for the rest of my life. I recommend you do as well.

HOW DO I DECIDE IF <u>NOW</u> IS THE RIGHT TIME TO HIRE

The more time you spend planning, the less scary or risky those big decisions (like hiring) feel. I want you to plan, but not to use "I'm planning" as an excuse to put it off for years.

"How do I decide if now is the right time to hire?", is a question I get asked a lot. It seems that a lot of owners I talk with – particularly new clinic owners – are always "preparing" to hire. They're always in the planning phase of hiring, but they never get around to doing it. They're always deciding over the right role, the right time, the right person, and so on, but they never actually *decide*.

Know this: there's a difference between *deciding* and *making a decision*. It's not uncommon for people to spend years in the *deciding* phase, yet it only takes a second to make a *decision*. To help me get out of the deciding phase and into the decision making phase, I use a simple framework. I call it my **Decision Framework**, and if I am ever stuck between a "rock and a hard place", uncertain about whether or not I need to hire, I'll often go to it.

Turn the page to see it…

PAUL'S HIRING DECISION FRAMEWORK

1. **WHAT IS THE UPSIDE OF HIRING SOMEONE?**

2. **WHAT IS THE LIKELIHOOD THAT IF I HIRE THE RIGHT PERSON, I WILL GET THE UPSIDE I WANT?**

3. **WHAT IS THE DOWNSIDE OF HIRING? (I.E. WHAT WILL IT COST ME?)**

4. **WHAT IS THE CHANCE OF GETTING HIRING WRONG? (I.E. 20%)**

5. **CAN I LIVE WITH THE DOWNSIDE?**

Let's walk through it together…

I'll use the scenario of hiring a front desk person whose salary is going to cost me $36,000. As you go through this it is important not to overthink any of it. Just follow the exercise and write down what comes into your head as you do. At the end, you'll have a decision made.

1. WHAT IS THE UPSIDE?

The first question is I have to ask myself is, "what will I get out of this hire?" In other words, how will this hire help improve my business? What problems, that are currently costing me time and money, will this person solve? What revenue will this person bring in that I am currently losing? It could be something like $100,000. If you're constantly missing calls or patients are dropping off, this number wouldn't be that far off. So, the upside of getting this decision right is $100,000 (because lost revenue would be saved).

2. WHAT ARE THE CHANCES OF THEM HELPING ME TO SOLVE THAT PROBLEM?

This step is you looking at the odds of success of having the above problem solved. You are asking, "if I make this hire and I do it right, what are the odds that my problem will be solved?"

The answer could be something like an 80% chance of success. It's important to remember that in this question you are just asking yourself about the problem being solved, not about choosing the right candidate. If you choose the right candidate, will your problem be solved, and what are the chances of this happening?

3. WHAT IS THE DOWNSIDE?

The downside is a maximum of three months' salary (and perhaps a little headache or frustration if you hire a complete dummy). That is because the absolute worst that can happen is that the hire costs you no more than three months' salary.

Remember, all **employees come with a payment plan**. That means you are not hiring someone for $36,000; you are paying them $3,000 per month. Assuming you have done the legal side of the contract correctly, and you inserted a 90 days trial/probation period in there (consult a lawyer for exact terms and conditions in your state/town), then after 90 days, if the hire doesn't work out, you can both go your separate ways.

That means the downside of the decision (in this example) is, at worst, going to cost you $9,000. But realistically, it isn't even costing you that much. Even the least productive employee you could hire is going to be doing something to drive revenue for you – or free your time up to drive more of it yourself.

Basically, whatever the annual salary is you are going to be paying, divide it by 12 months and multiply that by three (months), and that'll tell you how much this decision could cost you if it goes wrong. In this case, it is $9,000.

4. WHAT ARE THE CHANCES OF THE DOWNSIDE HAPPENING?

Without a real hiring process the chances of the downside happening (you losing three months' salary) are 50-50. It is potluck. You might get on the right side of the decision, but there's just as much chance of it going wrong.

However, with a real hiring process in place (the one I am giving you in this book), the chances lower. You're never going to get it right first time, every time, but if you follow a process, we can lower the odds of the downside to, let's say, 20%.

5. CAN YOU LIVE WITH IT?

Once you know the worst-case scenario (three months wages), and the odds of it happening (20%), the next thing you are able to do is actually make a decision about those odds and their potential downside.

In this case, if you can live with a **20%** chance of losing **$9,000**, and you're willing to risk it for the chance of solving your problem (which could result in **$100,000** worth of revenue), and there's an **80%** chance of the desired outcome coming to fruition, then you go ahead and stop deciding and make the decision to hire. What is more, you're going to give it all your time and attention because you know it's the right decision.

There! The decision is made. Either it is time to hire – or it isn't.

And if the answer is "no", then you need to look more closely at your finances and money management. Get yourself a cushion of cash so that the loss is not as painful; so that you *can* live with the downside. As a general rule of thumb, having the equivalent of two to three months' salary worth of cash sitting in your bank would be a good position to be in when hiring.

CONSIDERATION #2: MONEY

The next part of the plan to consider is how much money you have sitting in the bank. As small business owners, we do not live in a world of unlimited budgets. And the faster you have to hire, the more money it is going to cost you. So, it helps to take into account how much money you do currently have. This has nothing to do with compensation (what you'll pay the employee), this is about how you will get in front of the candidates in the first place.

It takes money to get in front of people, and the faster you need to do it, the more it will cost you.

Think about it: if you need to employ someone right away because the person who is answering the phone has quit (or you fired them), then you are in urgent need of having the phone answered. That means you are more likely to have to go to recruitment agencies, those that have a list of candidates waiting to be interviewed the next day.

The problem is, they want big money to access that list.

If you are going to use them, it *is* going to cost you. But the decision is not made on price, but on the net difference between what you have to pay them and the cost of lost business (if the phone goes unanswered for a month while you start the process on your own).

For example, if you're currently losing $10,000 per week in business, and the recruiting agency wants $10,000 for a list of physical therapists looking for a job, you might be better off paying them! However, if you're prepared and you saw this coming – it was in the annual plan – then you're going to be ready for it, and therefore you won't be in a rush.

Being ready means, you can keep this money, and if you can avoid using an agency then you will be more profitable at the end of the year. Which is why it pays to have a hiring plan – and a regularly updated business plan that details your growth plans - and to always be hiring.

CONSIDERATION #3: COMPENSATION (HOW MUCH SHOULD YOU PAY THEM?)

The next thing to consider is, what do you pay them? It's the million-dollar question. You find someone that you like; someone who you think can solve your problems. You don't want to pay them too little, yet at the same time you don't want to pay them too much. You're counterbalancing.

There are a lot of ideas out there about how much you should pay someone, but the bottom line is this: the more attractive your compensation package is, the easier it is to hire the right people. If you are paying at market rate and you have no brand recognition, a situation which means people are not desperately wanting to work for you (like they want to work for Zappos or Facebook or Google), then it might take longer and require more money to recruit the right person.

This adds more weight to the argument that, as the owner of a business, you must be actively marketing in your community. The importance of growing a brand and becoming a recognized name in your community is not just important for attracting new patients, it is just as important for recruiting staff.

In my town I've become a recognized and familiar name. That's because of my published books, my newspaper columns, non-stop marketing in the local area, active social media presence, and so on. Paul Gough Physio Rooms has become a "famous" place in the small towns we occupy. What's more, we've become a place in which people want to come and work.

For example, our social media is mostly all about our staff. On our media channels, we showcase their personalities and the fun that our staff have at work every day. There's not a single week that goes by when someone doesn't get in touch to ask if there's a job going at my place, because to them "we seem like a great place to work". Now, I am not saying that is my go-to recruitment strategy, but I am saying it helps. I have people asking to work at my clinic even when I am not advertising jobs. Aside from keeping my staff on their toes, it lessens the likelihood that I'll have to spend money with recruitment firms or job sites.

So, not only is my personal and clinic brand being strengthened by our marketing, we're strengthening our position when it comes to recruitment, too.

HOW MUCH YOU CHARGE DICTATES HOW MUCH YOU CAN PAY

Something else that is important to consider when deciding how much to pay people is how much your patients are currently paying you. Said bluntly:

> *"Most clinics do not charge enough to provide the level of service that people want to pay for".*

What that means is that business owners will often set their fees/rates so low when they are starting out, that it makes attracting the best staff almost impossible later on.

Their new patient acquisition strategy is to be a "cheap enough" provider and hope that, because they are cheap, people will choose them over the more expensive competition. The fee they charge only just covers the price of staying in business, only allowing for a small take home salary at the end. The clinic owner becomes content and happy to "get by". In order to avoid losing what patients they've got, prices are kept low.

Fine. I get it. But the problem with this thinking is that the price is not set to factor in the cost of marketing and paying the right staff. As a result, the owner is then shackled with Holiday Inn type staff, whilst all the time hoping they're going to deliver Ritz-Carlton type service. Which of course, never occurs. You can deliver high quality service, with high quality outcomes – but not at low quality prices. Try to do it for long enough and you'll find yourself stuck or out of business.

Here's another way to look at it: if your front desk person is being paid $20,000, but is not converting inquires, is not stopping drop-off's, and is not being spoken about in patient conversations (to friends and families of your past patients, when your clinic is mentioned), then she is costing you $120,000 (one hundred thousand more in lost revenue – plus the salary).

If you paid $30,000 – an extra $10,000 – to get a more skilled person, even if that person brought in just half of that $120,000 (that the cheaper staff person is losing), you'd be $50,000 better off. Which do you want?

SALARY OR PAY-PER-PATIENT?

If the level of compensation is one thing to consider, so is the type of compensation. Let's talk about how you pay physical therapists. Is it better to pay them a fixed salary or to go "50/50" and split the fee per patient of everyone the therapist sees?

For full disclosure, I've done both. That means what I am about to tell you is my experience and not my theory. I've tested both options and can tell you, in no uncertain terms, that I'd never go back to giving my physical therapists a percentage of what they earn.

I don't care how many people do it – it is not the right way to grow a profitable business, and I'll explain why:

Think about how and why this situation happens in the first place. It's not out of choice – it is usually by necessity; there's more than enough work for one, but not quite enough cash to cover all of the salary of a second therapist. There's a lot of phone calls one week, but not as many the next. There is inconsistent lead flow, and when there's no predictable system for delivering new leads and patients it will feel risky to pay someone a full-time salary.

Having to find $60k, $70k, $80k, or more for your first hire is daunting at first. It can be very scary, and so the "logical" solution appears to be to take someone on via splitting fees. Everyone is going to make a bit more money without the owner having to take on any additional risk.

And it works – at first. It often starts ok, but it isn't long before the problems surface.

HOW YOUR PROFIT MARGINS <u>DROP</u> FOLLOWING THIS SPLIT FEE MODEL

For starters, what can and most likely will happen is that your clinic revenue will increase, but your profit margins will decrease. Here's why: after the time that you agree on the 50/50 split, your rent goes up, the gas, electric and other expenses rise, and yet the physical therapist (on a split of the fee) is walking home with the same amount of money.

As a "paid per patient" physical therapist, they are the only enterprise on earth not subject to a rise in expenses.

Worse, if you try to raise your rates, the therapist will likely push back, fearful of losing income if they can't convert at the new higher price. They might not want to, but your situation requires it as you need to raise the rates to cover your rising expenses.

Then there's a stalemate; there's rarely any progress. Tensions rise and it's not great for company culture. From now it is likely to be months and perhaps years of wanting them out – or living in fear that they'll leave and set up against you. Either of those two is no way to try to grow a business.

I've coached hundreds of business owners, and almost all of their staffing problems, headaches, and hassles come from staff not being as committed as the owner's would like them to be; part time or split fee staff are almost always the chief culprits.

Pay-per-patient leads to fighting between therapists who manipulate the schedule in their favor. It also leads to other problems when patients want to be seen on different days, yet that therapist isn't working then. I've seen arguments between front desk and therapist when 'pay-per-patient' therapists see their schedules are not full – and someone else's is. It really does cause a lot of unwanted problems in a business.

Here's another point that you must not overlook: as your clinic's name and recognition in the market place increases over time, so does your value in the market place. That is an asset that you've created. And as I've been taught, **income follows assets**. Having this increased brand recognition leads to more confidence and trust in people's decisions to choose you. When you get to this point you've got more demand than supply. You've achieved what I call "deal flow" (where more people want to hire you than you can accommodate). It is the ultimate position to be in for any business.

It is at this point that you can start to raise rates more easily and frequently, and as a business owner you'll see more profit coming to you more quickly.

However, when you have a 50-50 split with a therapist, he or she is getting half of that pay rise. That's not the way it should ever work. If your business is the sum of its parts (which is must be), then *all* of the things like marketing, front desk people, training, culture, trust, brand recognition, location etc., are also included in the decision for patients to hire you. That cannot be split 50-50. At best, the therapist may get a 5-10% bump, but to give them 50% of the new price is being disrespectful to all of the other parts of your business I've just described.

Take from my experience what you will, but at the very least, and after reading this, I hope you'll have more respect for <u>all</u> of the parts that make up your business. The worst number in business is one, and if you're feeling like you have to rely upon one superstar, and you're frightened to challenge that person in case you lose them, then that is highlighting problems elsewhere in the business. Fix them first.

THE MORE RISK YOU TAKE – THE MORE YOU SHOULD MAKE

I started with pay-as-you-play therapists, and now they're all salaried and I'd never go back. I did it to get going – but, I didn't stay there.

I learned the hard way that getting part time, or "50/50 split" staff involved in meetings, coaching sessions, weekly training, or even asking them to do "free" discovery visits (that are a vital bridge in the patient conversion process), is tough. And that is where it starts to really cost you.

I've heard countless stories of therapists involved in this model regularly taking home more than the clinic owners, and just in case you needed reminding, that is <u>not</u> the way it is supposed to be.

Business owners (you and I) are actually supposed to make the most money. That *is* the way it is supposed to be because you and I take the biggest risks. We take on the most stress and hassle, and it's our credit rating on the line if we're unable to meet the business loan or make rent.

I believe that as a business owner it is that burden and being able to live with that risk – and still make great decisions – is what you ultimately get paid for. The more risk and responsibility you can handle, the more of the money you will make.

Believe me, the big money that you make will, in the end, have little to do with how hard you work, how much you "hustle", or even how great of a clinician you are; it is all to do with shouldering risk and responsibility.

It took me a while to understand this; your income as a business owner is tied to risk and responsibility, as well as your ability to manage and live with that.

I had been "conditioned" by friends, family, and the media, all of whom will have you believe that the way to be successful is to "work harder". The problem is that most of the people who tell you the secret of success is to work hard, haven't actually achieved that much success themselves. Do not confuse a safe job, a 4-bedroom house, and two kids in private school with success. They're likely going to work every day hating what they do just to pay for those things. That is not success. It is stupidity.

Why do they stay in a job they hate? It is because it is too risky to leave it. It is because they can't, or don't, want to have the responsibility of paying ten peoples' wages at the end of the month whilst having to make rent.

When you think about what we business owners really do, it is take the risk and assume levels of responsibility that the other 90% of people in society, those who want a safe job, could never do.

True story: I once bought a black, soft top Porsche Carrera 911 S4. I was 28. I was making a decent sum of money at the time, filling almost every single position in the clinic. I was a full-time therapist, marketer, sales person, operations manager – you name it, I was doing it (…it was before I knew the value of hiring good staff). But, I was too busy working to find time to spend the money I was making; this was a time that was pre-children, and I had nothing else to spend it on, so I thought I would treat myself to a new car.

When I bought the car I had a lot of people commenting that "business must be doing well". I told anyone who asked about it (staff included) that I was only able to buy the car because of the crap, hassle, stress, and big, bold decisions that I make each day running my clinic.

I told them that the more of *that* I take, the more money I make.

I did not come to be in a position of buying a $100k car because of the lower backs I fixed, or hamstring strains I diagnosed, no matter how good I was at it.

This risk and responsibility thing are directly proportional to your success, and what is more, this should never be forgotten as you take on staff or are ever fearful of taking home a huge salary. You and I do the stuff that 90% of the world does not want to do. Job creation and business building is risky, and it consumes your thoughts 24/7. As a result, you should get to live a little differently from the other 90%. That's the deal.

If you want to make more, go for it. You deserve it. If you want to increase the rates at your clinic because you need to <u>fund a new Yacht</u> for you and your family to relax in on the lake at weekends – do it. Don't hold back or try to hide from it with some crappy excuse about the rent going up, thereby forcing you to raise rates.

Instead, look your staff firmly in the eye when they ask why you're raising rates (again) and tell them that "it's because you've seen a better version of the boat you're currently driving on a weekend, <u>and you want to upgrade</u>."

What is more, tell them it's available anytime they want to borrow it…

My point is this: hiring people is risky. You will never get away from that. But the more risk you take (calculated of course), the more you will make. And, don't let anyone *ever* tell you that you don't deserve to make more money than your staff. You do. In todays "PC" world, the masses are ganging up on us business owners and trying very hard to have you believe that you don't, or shouldn't, be doing it. As if somehow entrepreneurship is evil and because you want to make money, you're greedy.

Like I said at the very start of this book – **the majority is always wrong.**

Know your worth. Never lose sight of what it is that you do, and bill accordingly for it. And if you're still thinking of taking on part time staff or "splitting the fee", my advice would be to make sure that you get the biggest chunk of the upside to factor in all of the expenses that will increase. At best, start there – but don't stay there.

Anyhow, that's the entire hiring plan covered and one or two other big questions to-boot. Come with me to chapter six and I'll help you to *"establish the financial metric of success"* for your next hire.

If you can't answer the question of "what is this hire going to be worth to me", why are you even doing it?…

6

STEP 2/6:
HOW TO ESTABLISH THE FINANCIAL METRIC OF SUCCESS FOR A NEW HIRE

This one's a short chapter: if Step 1 in the hiring process is *Create the Hiring Plan*, Step 2 is getting clear on what success actually looks like for you, **financially.**

As business owners, what we really do is multiply capital (your money) by leveraging assets (your staff and marketing system). If I am hiring someone and I'm going to be paying him or her $25,000, I want to know what my return will be.

Before you get deep into the hiring process you want to know how much a hire is going to be worth to you. If you can see what you stand to make by hiring (or what you're going to lose if you don't do it), then you're much more likely to be fully committed to the process and avoid all of the mistakes we covered in chapter 2.

This is called <u>establishing the financial metric of success</u>. You are answering the question, "how would I know if this was a successful hire?"

Think about that question for a moment... I suspect you'll be tempted to write down things like the characteristics or qualities in the candidate that you are hoping to find. But, that is not what we're talking about here. We want to know about the possible financial implications that this decision would have on your business. Is the risk worth the reward?

To my regret, this is a step I inserted much later on than all the rest in my hiring process. And yet, it has proved to be one of the most helpful. It is the process of working out what the financial return on your asset needs to be in order to make it worthwhile.

Remember, the people in your business are assets. And any investment you make in any asset needs to produce a return; that is what assets are supposed to do. If it is true that income follows assets, which it is, then how much income needs to follow *this asset* to tell you that you've invested in a good one?

The clarity that this little exercise will bring you is astounding. And, if you find yourself caught in the "shall I" or "shall I wait" way of thinking about hiring, this is another way of overcoming the doubt or procrastination.

What is more, I've found that every time I've done this exercise I actually become more confident about hiring, as I can see what this hire is going to be worth to me.

This goes way beyond defining a successful hire as "having the right qualifications", or "being the right cultural fit" – it is about the return that business will get if the person you hire does everything that you need them to do. Remember, this is an Outcome Based Hiring System.

This part of the process involves two aspects; let me talk you through them both:

PART 1: WHAT PROBLEM ARE YOU SOLVING?

I've mentioned this before – you need to know this. Now I am going to make it real for you and ask that you write it down.

Let's do this exercise together for your upcoming or next immediate hire. Think about your business's current biggest problem. What is it? Most people will say it's the symptom of the problem. That might be something like "we have a conversion issue to sort out", or, "we have a drop off issue", or, "we need more leads."

When you know what the symptom is (the thing that is causing you to feel like you need to hire), write it down here now:

Now, define what the real problem is that you've got. (Is it that you don't have the right person? Is it that you don't have enough of the right people? Is it a marketing message issue? Is it a lack of focus on the patient experience?)

And finally, write down if this falls under a retention issue or an acquisition issue?

Now that you know what the real problem is that you're solving, let's move on to part two:

PART 2: GET FINANCIAL CLARITY

SCENARIO 1: HIRING FRONT DESK PERSON

I'll walk you through this first, then you can do it for yourself after.

For this one, I am going to use a common scenario that happens too often in many clinics: the phone is ringing with inquiries, but it is not being answered. Either there is no one there to answer it at all, or everyone is too busy treating patients.

Having done step 1, I conclude that my biggest problem is that we have a retention issue; we are losing patients that are calling yet not scheduling appointments. I am estimating that we're missing out on <u>one</u> phone call per day that, if we answered, and had the time to speak to that person correctly, would lead to an additional <u>3 new patients per week.</u>

The patient is worth $1000 to me, so I am currently losing $3000 per week. That is approximately $13-$14,000 per month. That means this front desk hire *could* be worth as much as $150,000 in revenue *if* I get the hire right. That is my financial metric of success.

The cost of the hire is going to be about $25,000, which means I could stand to gain a 1:6 return on my money. That means, for every $1 I spend on this person's salary, I will get $6 back. That is a very good return on your money… the odds are in your favor.

Now, of course, I am estimating. But, I am using this as a framework from which I can make a better, more educated, more informed decision. As a happy by-product, simply seeing this number in black and white, on paper, also instantly makes it feel less risky. It gives me more confidence because it confirms that I really do need to hire.

As an aside, what I have just described is likely happening to many of the tens of thousands of people who will read this book.

So many will have a phone ringing, yet, one that is not being answered properly (if at all). And that alone is the reason they're not making as much money as they would like. A lot of clinic owners will try to keep their admin costs down, thinking they are saving money. And, as a result, they are most likely losing more than they're saving. It is a crazy way to run a business, and yet so many do it.

Here's a thought: the reason they don't have the money to pay the people they need is because the people who are calling are not converting - they're not converting because no one is taking the time to explain why they should pay the fees or what they're actually paying for. Maybe if someone did that, patients would feel more comfortable and confident about paying? It is not rocket science.

You'll always get what you tolerate in this life, and if your front desk person is having to put more than one person on hold per day or is missing just one call per day that goes to voicemail, then there's a chance that this scenario is already happening to you – and it's time to hire.

Next, let's take a look at how it might play out for a physical therapist...

SCENARIO 2: HIRING A PHYSICAL THERAPIST

In the case of a physical therapist, I'm projecting that the current number of inquiries we're losing is something like five patients per week. And if my average patient spends $1,000, that means I am currently losing around $22,000 per month._That is close to $250,000 per year.

So, in this case, the hire should be worth $250,000 (less their salary) to my gross profit. With this type of financial clarity I can then decide what I am willing to pay. If the right candidate wants $5,000 more than the second best candidate, I am more confident about paying it. I can see what the financial windfall looks like, assuming that they hit all of their targets (something we will come to in the next chapter).

Now that I've walked you through it, here is the framework for you to do this exercise yourself – turn the page to get going...

What is the problem?

_____

How much is that costing you each day, right now?

_____

How much is that costing you per month?

_____

How much is that costing you per year?

_____

How much do you estimate you stand to make per year if you solved it?

_____

What is the cost of solving it (i.e. employee salary)?

_____

What is the net difference that you stand to gain by hiring (i.e. what you stand to make minus salary cost)?

_____

The figure above is your _financial metric of success._

The question is, are you happy to proceed? Is it worthwhile? Do you still want to hire? Like I said earlier, doing this exercise is designed to get you clear on what success looks like. What is possible for you to get in return for hiring this person? What is your return on expenditure likely to be? Can you pay a little more than you thought to get the one you want? Do this before the recruitment phase starts and you'll know.

And like we said in Chapter 5, *Create The Hiring Plan*, what you are able to pay can sometimes make the difference in getting the best person or not. Not always I might add, but it sure does give you more options. More money doesn't solve everything, but I am yet to be in a situation where having more money didn't give me a <u>distinct advantage.</u>

So, after doing that exercise, and if you are happy with the financial return, let's move on to the next step. Here we're going to create what I call the *Success Description*; it will act as your "north star", your "guiding light" throughout the rest of the process. It will ensure that you select an A Player to join your team.

Turn over the page and let's get to work on creating it…

7

STEP 3/6:
HOW TO CREATE YOUR SUCCESS DESCRIPTION (OUTCOMES, TASK, MEASURE, SKILLS)

Step 1 of the process is about *creating a hiring plan*. You wouldn't book a vacation without having a plan, and you shouldn't be making a hire without one either. The plan involves factoring in time, money, and compensation.

Step 2 is asking yourself, "what does success look like?", and putting down on paper what the *financial metric of success* of your hire is. This gives you a yardstick of success; an objective view of performance that lifts you out of relying upon gut feeling or emotions.

This brings us to **Step 3**; because you now know what success looks like, you can accurately create a description of the person that you're looking for; the person who will achieve that level of success for you.

This is what I call the Success Description. It is a profile of the person who you want to hire, one who is able to reach the outcome that you want to achieve.

The Success Description is a move away from the traditional "job description" that is the norm when it comes to recruitment. With the traditional job description there is no focus on achieving an outcome, and there's often a vague understanding of what success even looks like. Skills are confused with features (such as "must be hard working") and, more often than not, job descriptions are focused on finding someone with experience. Which, you now know, doesn't always guarantee a great candidate.

I've said it many times; you can always spot an employer who doesn't really know what they're looking for – they'll advertise for someone with "experience".

They think it is a safe bet, but it rarely works out that way. They're often just more experienced at stuff you don't need them or want them to do.

This Success Description is a physical document that you'll create, and then have with you, throughout the entirety of the rest of the hiring process. When I am in hiring mode, this document is never too far away from me; it is either in my hand or on my desk right until the decision is made.

The printed PDF acts as my guide for the questions I will ask, reminds me what skills and competencies I am looking for, as well as re-enforces what problem the people I am talking to will be solving for me. It's easy to forget or get distracted during the interview, and this document stops me from doing so.

What is more, when the Success Description is complete, I can use it to create the job ad that'll I'll soon be posting (that we'll cover in chapter 8).

The Success Description is broken up into five parts, and I'm going to walk you through all of them. To help you follow along, here's what the shell of one looks like: (turn over the page to see it)

FIG.7 — FRAMEWORK OF THE SUCCESS DESCRIPTION SHOWING THE FIVE PARTS

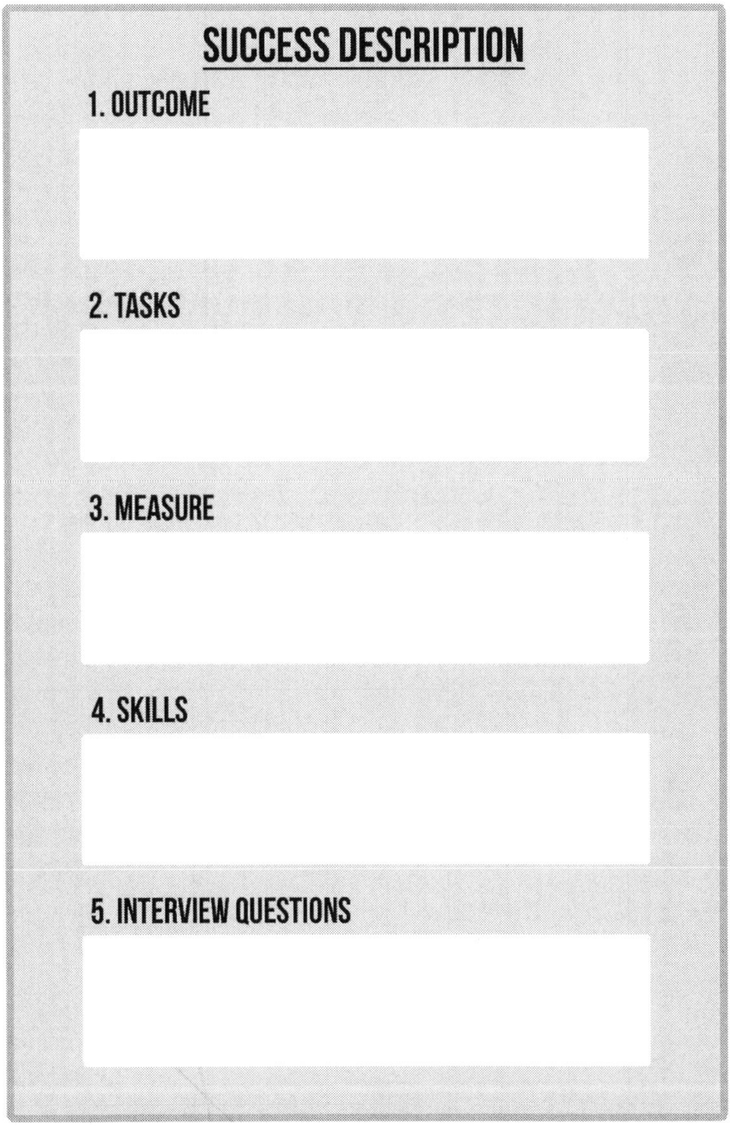

SUCCESS DESCRIPTION

1. OUTCOME

2. TASKS

3. MEASURE

4. SKILLS

5. INTERVIEW QUESTIONS

> **DOWNLOAD YOUR DONE-FOR-YOU SUCCESS DESCRIPTIONS**
>
> You can download this worksheet by going to
> **www.paulgough.com/hiring-resource**
>
> You can also get a completed example of this *Success Description* as well. I've included in the PDF a filled-out **Success Description** for a physical therapist, as well as the exact *Success Description* that I used to fill a front desk role at my own clinic – while writing this book.
>
> Before we move on, I strongly recommend that you get and download the PDF document so that you can follow along with me in this chapter. You'll be able to see clearly all that I am about to describe, as well as where the relevant sections fit into your *Success Description*. Do this by going to:
>
> **www.paulgough.com/hiring-resource**

HOW TO CREATE A SUCCESS DESCRIPTION

I break this up into five sections, four of which make up the Outcomes Based Hiring Success Triangle introduced in chapter 1; Here are the five parts to it:

1. The Big Outcome

2. The Tasks

3. Measurable Standards

4. Skills/Competencies Required

5. Questions To Ask At The Interview

Let's look at each one in depth – we'll walk through it together with examples for both a front desk person and a physical therapist:

1. THE BIG OUTCOME

This is the one paragraph summary of the essence of the job. This is where you write down what the core purpose of the role is in conjunction with the problem you are solving. This is about you understanding why you need to hire someone in the first place. We've covered this in "theory" so far, and now you're going to write it down. So, get ready to put pen to paper and write no more than one paragraph, clearly explaining why the role exists.

EXAMPLE OF THE BIG OUTCOME FOR A FRONT DESK/ADMIN PERSON

Let me help you out by giving you an example of what the 'big outcome' for a **traditional front desk person** could be. It might go something like this:

> "To grow the revenue of the clinic by retaining the patients that we have. This person will also convert any new interest that comes to us as a result of the goodwill or word of mouth that already exists in our community. Doing this will involve developing a deep and meaningful relationship with our patients, spending time getting to know each one personally, and answering their concerning questions about physical therapy. We need this person to create the type of experience that customers can't wait to come back to, will be happy to pay for, and be just as happy to tell others about."

THE BIG OUTCOME FOR A PHYSICAL THERAPIST

And, here's what the 'big outcome' for a **physical therapist** could look like:

> "To grow the revenue of the clinic by ensuring that all of our patients complete their recommended plan of care. Doing this means they are more likely to get the outcome they want, will receive full value for money, and in turn will be happy to have chosen us. This will turn them into lifelong, raving fans as well as reliable referral sources, as they mention our name to anyone considering physical therapy."

For the 'big outcome' to be meaningful, it has to be written in a very simple and easy to understand way. With that said, here's an example of **what not to do:**

> "The physical therapist is to provide an exceptional standard of clinical care by following the latest and most up-to-date research guidelines. They will do this whilst having excellent knowledge of the newest treatment modalities. In addition, the physical therapist will simultaneously maximize patient satisfaction as well as contribute to the excellent atmosphere and professional standards in the clinic."

All of those things are features, not outcomes. You can't measure, monitor or track the performance of features. This is where most business owners go wrong; they don't just make the mistake in hiring, but also in their marketing. They describe things like "years in business", or "expert qualifications", as though they are benefits. They are not. They are features that go into achieving the benefit that the customer wants. The customer buys benefits, not features. It's the same for hiring - you should hire people for outcomes, not features. Therefore, you must be talking more about benefits and less about features in this process.

2. THE TASKS

So now that you know what the 'big outcome' is, the next thing you have to do is consider the tasks that are required to achieve that outcome - what needs to be done or completed by this person in order to achieve the outcome?

Let's take a look at some examples of what those tasks could be:

TASKS FOR A TRADITIONAL FRONT DESK/ADMIN PERSON

Remember, my definition of the traditional front of house person is the guy or girl who is sitting at your front desk in reception, answering the phone from hot prospects, past patients, and their referrals. They also meet and greets patients as they come through the door. What you are doing here is asking:

"What does this front desk person need to do and achieve in order to bring success in the role?"

It could be things like:

- Communicate the value of our services (in person and on the phone) and be able to explain how what we do is worth the price we are asking.

- Successfully handle price objections.

- Hold a lengthy (at least 15-20 minute) conversation with new patients on the phone, ensuring patients are committed and bought into our service.

- Provide an exceptional waiting room environment for our patients, one that they'll look forward to coming back to.

- Ensure that people who call and request appointments are placed on schedule (and understand the true time and cost commitment involved in physical therapy before they arrive).

- Ensure people show up excited for their first appointment after scheduling.

- Communicate with patients before, during, and after appointments in order to ensure that satisfaction is being achieved.

- Ensure that all invoices are raised on time, every time, and are sent to the appropriate person (in house or externally).

- Organize and plan all schedules – maximizing efficiency and revenue for the clinic.

- Foster deep relationships with patients, ensuring NPS (Net Promoter Score) hits agreed levels.

- Develop and regularly update the procedure library so that every aspect of the role is documented, ensuring it can be achieved by anyone else in the business.

Those are examples of things that I want my new front desk person to achieve for me. I am highlighting and stressing "me" on purpose, as they may not be exactly what you want your front desk person to do – but, those are the type of things I expect my front desk staff to do for me.

You don't have to copy my tasks word for word; just copy the thought process and how I came to the conclusion of what I want. Notice that what I am asking for is a far cry from the usual things you see in a job description. Those types of things include "being professional and friendly", "owning the department", or "being reliable and committed". You don't need to ask an A Player to bring those features to work – they come as standard.

TASKS FOR A PHYSICAL THERAPIST

Remember, physical therapists are in retention. They sit in the operations department of your business and their job is to <u>deliver on the promise made by the marketing message and the sales team</u>.

With that in mind, here's an example of the tasks I would expect of any physical therapist that *I* am hiring.

It could be things like:

- Communicate with patients in a way that allows them to confidently make the right decision about the plan of care you suggest.

- Ensure that patients achieve their clinical and health/lifestyle outcomes (in the time frame you set).

- Develop a mutually beneficial relationship that benefits both the patient and the clinic.

- Communicate the value of our service with the fee/price that the patient will need to pay to access it.

- Ensure that patients remain excited about the prospect of coming for physical therapy (and remain committed to the treatment plan that you suggest).

- Provide a high level of customer care that will cause patients to want to come back frequently (and tell their friends and family about us as well).

- Ensure that patients coming for free taster/discovery sessions convert to a first evaluation (when appropriate).

- Ensure that patients agree to a plan of care that will help them hit their health goals.

- Ensure that patients complete a full plan of care (as agreed in the first session).

- Ensure that clinical notes are kept up-to-date, accurate, and completed in the agreed time frame needed for the clinic to complete the billing.

- Participate in, contribute to, and help to develop the in-house educational training program that is provided to all physical therapists.

These are the benefits of me hiring them. They are the problems that I want solving. And these are things that the physical therapist will be responsible for, once they are hired.

3. MEASURABLE OUTCOMES

Which brings us to the next part – measuring. The Hiring Success Triangle is about outcomes, tasks, and skills centered around measuring.

So, the next (and possibly the most important) step is to turn those tasks into standards that you can measure – measurable outcomes. What you measure will be used to recognize when you need to coach this person to improve their performance if it has dipped.

As a leader of a business, I firmly believe that one of my most important roles is to coach and optimize the performance of my team. If I want improvements from my team, then I have to know where they currently are before I start. I can only do that if I measure.

What's more, you will only achieve a world-class team of people in your clinic if you can hold them accountable for their performance. Without measurable outcomes or accountability, it is human nature for standards to drop. That's why this is a vital step in the hiring process.

As a general rule, I try not to set more than 3-5 measurable outcomes. If you are not careful, you'll spend more time looking at data than running your clinic. Think of these measurable outcomes as a warning light that appears on the dashboard of your car; when it goes off, you know something is wrong. You're not 100% sure what it is, so you start asking a few questions of the right person in order to determine what it might be.

The same thing is needed in business. Having these measurable outcomes is your version of the warning light alerting you to something that is not quite right. Only this is not what is wrong with your car – it's what's wrong with your business. They are signals telling you that you should look a little deeper at what your staff are doing. Or, as is most often the case, what they are *not* doing.

So, let's take a look at what some examples could be for a front desk person and physical therapist…

MEASURABLE OUTCOMES FOR A FRONT DESK/ADMIN

Here's an example of how I would quantify a front desk person's performance, using examples from four of those tasks described in the previous section:

1. Conversion from incoming/warm inquiry to paying patient greater than 80%

2. Arrival for first appointment greater than 95%

3. Re-schedule 90% of drop-offs within 30 days

4. Physical Therapist utilization ratio greater than 85% (but no more than 95%)

MEASURABLE OUTCOMES – PHYSICAL THERAPIST

That's how you would do it for a front desk person, next, let's take a look at how you might create objective measurements for a physical therapist.

Now that I know what I want the physical therapist to do (tasks), I am able to quantify the 3-5 most important parts of their job as well; the things that if they get right for me, means my business is a boat sailing into the sunset (and not one sinking in the harbor). Here are five examples of how you could make their tasks measurable:

1. Conversion ratio from free taster/discovery visit to first evaluation greater than 80%

2. Conversion from first session to full plan of care greater than 80%

3. Completed plan of care ratio greater than 95%

4. Less than 1% of claims denied due to inaccurate note taking/filing

5. Net Promoter Score (NPS) of 8/10

Think about these outcomes for a moment; if you hired a physical therapist and you monitored only these five things, I'd be pretty sure that you'd either be happy with the results (and want to keep this person), or, you'd be moving them on if training/coaching didn't improve the results. Either way, you're in a better position and your business is going to be stronger for doing it.

Again, to get to these measurable outcomes, I simply started with a list of important tasks (listed in section 2), and I then prioritized them to the 4-5 that I believe to be the most critical to the role - the tasks that if they just got those four things right, would make it easier to be successful in my business.

All numbers in business are important, but there are always some numbers that are more important than others. That is what we're doing here – finding the most important ones to track. It's called prioritizing, and that in and of itself is a skill.

I call these numbers "critical drivers" because they are the critical numbers that will drive my company's results. While knowing KPI's and metrics are vital, I prefer to focus more on the critical drivers; if you get the critical drivers right, the KPI's take care of themselves.

Examples of KPI's are things like total revenue and profit. In other words, things that happen after the month has ended. I don't like finding out how my business has performed when it is too late to do anything about it. It's like a manager of a basketball team only being able to watch the replay of the games his team plays in. There's no way to make the tactical changes or substitutions that might have stopped the loss.

'Critical drivers' are known as 'leading indicators' of performance; they are things that you can change before they appear as a KPI (sales or profit). Monitor the critical drivers well enough and you won't have to worry about your revenue or profit, because they'll be where you want, as you will have made necessary changes ahead of time. It's a radically different way of running your business that really does work.

When you know what the measurable standards are, it's easy for you to:

a. Hire someone knowing what you need them to do (clarity on the goal)

b. Hold them accountable for achieving it (the primary role of a leader)

c. Coach/train to improve their performance when it dips (which it will from time to time)

Here's a key point to remember: I'm not saying that these exact numbers or standards are going to be right for <u>you</u>. What I am doing is explaining the framework that I use to come to the conclusions of what they need to look like for my clinic – so that you can create your own.

You can and should use the same way of thinking about this as me and come to your own conclusion of what these figures need to look like in order to hit your targets.

Don't obsess over the exact numbers – they are guides. The very fact that you're even spending some time doing this has already given you a better chance of success with hiring. Doing the exercise is more important than the number. Believe me when I say that by doing this you are definitely ahead of 99.9% of owners in our profession. Most would never dream of measuring their staff's performance (for fear of what they would find!), let alone know how to do it.

HOW TO TRACK THESE THINGS

Now after all of that, I suspect you're thinking, "all of this sounds great Paul, but how do you actually track these things?" Well, let me explain...

First of all, you need to accept that yes, it will take some time. You are going to spend time to save time. In an ideal world you are not the one inputting or monitoring the data. You are the one analyzing what the data is telling you. Big difference. Your job is to turn the information on the spreadsheet into knowledge about your clinic's performance.

I have my finance guy input the data for me, but it could be done by anyone. My tip is to do it yourself the first time so that you know how the mechanics of it work. Once you've done that, teach someone else to do it. It'll take you a few hours to teach your staff, and then you should be spending 40-60 minutes per week drawing conclusions from the data you are looking at. It really isn't as complicated as you might think.

For example, let's say you're tracking something like the number of people who converted from a discovery/taster session (the term I used to describe a free first visit). Of course, this would be a number you would be measuring for a physical therapist. To make sure they're doing a good job with converting, you want to know how many people your therapists saw at a discovery session took the next step and paid for a full consultation. This is called the conversion ratio.

To find it, you would look back at the last ten discovery visit sessions and check the number of people who said yes to booking a paid-for first session. It's a manual exercise, and you're looking within a set time frame of the last seven days, as an example.

Whatever it is, keep that time frame consistent. If you are looking for an 80% conversion ratio as your standard, then you need to see that eight of those ten people (or more) said yes and moved on to the next step.

If the number was seven or less, the target is not being hit. And if that were happening to me I would be talking to the therapist and finding out where the gaps are in his or her skill set. I'd then set about working with them to fill that gap and coaching them to see an improvement.

With that in mind, let's move on to the next part:

4. SKILLS AND COMPETENCIES NEEDED

The fourth aspect of the Success Description to consider is, "what skills and competencies are needed to reach the measurable outcomes that you've just created?"

The definition of skill" is "the ability to do something well". And, the definition of a "competency" is "the ability to do something successfully and efficiently".

That's something very important to consider; it's one thing being able to do something well, but does it take the person five times as long as someone else to do it? As clinics grow one of the reasons is they become less profitable is they get less efficient. Sure, the staff hired get stuff done – but if it takes longer than it should you'll end up hiring more people than you really need to come with the back log of work. Doing that increases your expenses and makes you less profitable than you could be.

Now that you know what each one is, let's consider what those skills and competencies need to be for each role in order to hit the outcomes that you're looking for. We'll look at a front desk person first.

SKILLS AND COMPETENCIES FOR A FRONT DESK PERSON

Here's an example of 12 skills or competencies that I might look for when trying to hire a front desk person. These are the things that they're going to have to do very well in order to be successful in the role.

For example:

1. Be able to hold meaningful conversations with prospective patients on the phone for longer than 20 minutes (empathy).

2. Be able to answer all questions asked on the phone in such a way that increases the likelihood that the person asking, will want to become a customer (insightful and knowledgeable).

3. Recall names and faces of patients, making all of our patients feel welcomed and remembered.

4. Provide a warm and welcoming greeting to patients when they arrive in the clinic (experience).

5. Organization and planning – plans, organizes, schedules and budgets in an efficient, productive manner. (Focuses on key priorities).

6. Follow through on commitments - lives up to verbal and written agreements regardless of personal cost.

7. Demonstrates an ability to quickly and proficiently understand and absorb new information.

8. Attention to detail - does not let important details slip through the cracks.

9. Persistence - demonstrates tenacity and willingness to go the distance to get something done.

10. Proactivity - acts without being told what to do. (Brings new ideas to the company).

11. Alertness – are they able to spot potential referral situations or opportunities for the sale of other products and services?

12. Resourceful – not everything always goes according to plan on front desk. How do they react when the internet connection is down or the phone line is cut off during a storm? Business has to carry on, and I want them to be more resourceful than complain of a lack of resources…

They don't have to be these things exactly. Although they are an accurate representation of the skills that I am looking for when I hire a front of house person. That's because all of these things, if done well, would significantly improve the chance of our patients being retained. And that is precisely the reason they were hired.

This part takes on even more importance when you come to the interview section of the process. "What questions do I ask in an interview?" is something everyone seems to want to know. Well, the answer is to ask questions that allow you find proof of the skills and competencies you need. The ones you've just listed above.

For example, if you are looking for someone who can "hold meaningful conversations with prospective patients on the phone for longer than 20 minutes", then <u>ask</u> for proof that they've got this particular skill.

Instead of asking random questions like, "what are your hobbies and interests?", you can instead ask for proof of specific situations where the candidate you are interviewing has previously demonstrated that particular skill - being able to put patients at ease is a skill, and to find out if the candidate has this skill I might ask this question:

"Tell me about a time when you had to talk to a nervous customer on the phone for more than 20 minutes – why were they nervous/skeptical, what did you do to make them more confident, and how did it end?"

Personally, I prefer to know that they have already done the type of thing that I am going to need them to do. If this is the first time at the rodeo it's going to cost me a lot of time teaching them how to ride. I'm not a huge fan being the first one to teach someone a new skill or competency. I much prefer to inherit someone with the skill and then work with them to optimize it. That's the nirvana that we are shooting for with hiring. And that's the difference I'm teaching you in this book. I can tell you from experience that it's much easier for a business owner to optimize a skill that is already there than to train from scratch.

This is also where experience and skills get confused; just because someone has done a "reception job" and answered the phone for 20 years, doesn't mean they've got this particular skill.

When you understand that it is possible for someone without experience in your role – to have the skills required of your role - it opens up the candidate pool considerably. There are a lot of roles out there where people are using the skills you need which are easily transferable to your role. Transferable skills do exist and it is possible for someone who has worked in for example an account managers role at a call center to end up as a superstar in a sales or nurture role at your clinic. It is possible for someone who has been a general manager in retail to become a world class general manager of a physical therapy clinic. All it takes is for you to understand what those skills are you need.

Next, let's look at the type of skills and competencies needed by a physical therapist to do his or her job successfully:

SKILLS AND COMPETENCIES FOR A PHYSICAL THERAPIST

For example, these could be:

1. Be able to communicate with patients in such a way that they can understand why the suggested plan of care is the best solution to solve their problem.

2. Communicate with patients in a way that they can see value in the plan of care being put forward to them in exchange for their time and money.

3. Willing and able to spot when a patient may be disillusioned or confused with their progress (and likely to drop off).

4. To be able to communicate in such a way that the patient can confidently say "yes" to a full plan of care.

5. To be able to engage with and connect with patients on a personal level that goes way beyond a clinical outcome.

6. Demonstrates an understanding of what the causes are – and solutions – that could lead to a patient dropping off schedule.

7. Demonstrates a willingness to be held accountable for performance.

8. Ability to thrive in an environment where measurement is the driving force behind progress.

Knowing the skills I am looking for, here's an example of a question I might ask when looking for one of those skills in my candidates:

"Tell me about a time when you recognized a patient who was disillusioned with their progress in PT – how did you spot it, what did you do about it to keep them on schedule, and how did it end?"

The question is purposeful and focused on the problem you want solving - losing patients. By asking this question you are getting closer to hiring someone who demonstrates the skills needed to solve the problem you've got.

5. THE QUESTIONS TO ASK

This brings us to the final part of the Success Description where you will list your interview questions. You can only list your questions when you know what you're looking for, which is why you've got to go through this process first before you can consider what you might ask. Doing the work to get to this point is important and that's because the quality of the questions really does dictate the quality of the answers you'll get.

You could say that everything so far had to happen just to get you to this point of knowing precisely what to ask.

Asking the right questions is ultimately what determines how you'll discover if the person is the one you need. Are they able to answer in a way that clearly demonstrates proof that they got the right skills and values you're looking for? Only by asking the right questions will you ever know.

Asking the right questions also takes you straight to the heart of the big problem in hiring; confusing personality with values. The two are not the same. When personality is mentioned it should really be re-classified as values. It's their values that determine how good of a cultural fit they are – not their personality. What people value is significantly more important than their personality. No one ever got fired for having a bad personality. They got fired because they didn't want to put the teams needs before their own. That's a value issue - it is out of sync with the owners values and those of the business.

There's going to be a lot more on the type of questions you should ask – both for skill and value – when we get to Chapter 10 (The Interview). But for now, I want you to realize where all of this is going: I am showing you a logical framework that if you follow, leads you to asking the right questions of the right candidates. The answers will give you the data to create a profile that you will try to match up against the profile of the person you're looking for. When they match up, you will make that person the job offer.

The blank version of the success description allows you to start writing questions directly underneath the skills and competencies you're looking for. We'll come back to this section in Chapter 10. Download it here: **www.paulgough.com/book-resource.**

WHAT ABOUT THE OTHER ROLES IN YOUR CLINIC?

In this chapter we've covered in-depth two examples on how to write your Success Description for a front desk/admin person and a physical therapist. But what about the other roles you might want to fill in marketing, sales and finance?

Well, you'll follow the exact same steps as we've just been through. What I suggest you do is print off a Success Description template for each, refer back to this chapter, then fill them out for the roles following the framework I've given you.

To help you, here's a couple of ideas of the things you could be measuring in three different roles:

- **Marketing** - acquire 5 new leads per month from our 3 lead generators (Facebook, Google and Newspaper Ads)

- **Sales/Nurture** – convert 1:3 cold leads to a discovery visit

- **Finance** – Accounts receivable days total no more than 30 days and never more than one month's operating expenses

A QUICK RE-CAP

Here's a quick summary of where we're up to:

At this point, all you are doing is putting down on paper (in three sections) what the **big outcome** is you want to achieve and what **tasks** are required to meet that outcome. This creates a measurable standard so that you know if the outcomes you set are being achieved. You can then consider what **skills** the person must have to do it for you. This allows you to get to the position of being able to ask the right questions, therefore getting the right answers.

This part of the process is being done by you, for you - it absolutely must be done by you and cannot be abdicated in anyway. It is going to take you about one or two hours to do it, but once you've done it that first time, you've got it for life. The next time you go to fill the same role you'll only need to make one or two alterations.

Be sure to use the worksheets and examples that I've provided to create your own Success Description for your upcoming hire. Get them all from here if you haven't done so already: **www.paulgough.com/hiring-resource**

You'll be pleased to know that we've done most of the hard work now. For the remainder of the Outcomes Based Hiring Process you can draw on much of the content in the Success Description; this content includes choosing the interview questions, creating the job ad, and posting it!

And that's what we're going to do next: *Create the Job Ad*. But not just any job ad... one that attracts the right quantity and quality of candidates who you'll soon start to interview.

Turn the page over and let's get going with *Creating the Job Ad*, we're up to part four in the six-part process.

8

• •

STEP 4/6: HOW TO CREATE YOUR JOB AD

Now that you've created the *Success Description*, the next thing to do is create the *job ad*. This is the "magnet" that will attract the right candidates, those with the right skills to perform the tasks required in order to achieve the **outcome** you need from the role. Those three things, centered around measurable standards, make up the ***Outcomes Based Hiring Success Triangle*** that I spoke to you about in the last chapter:

FIG.8

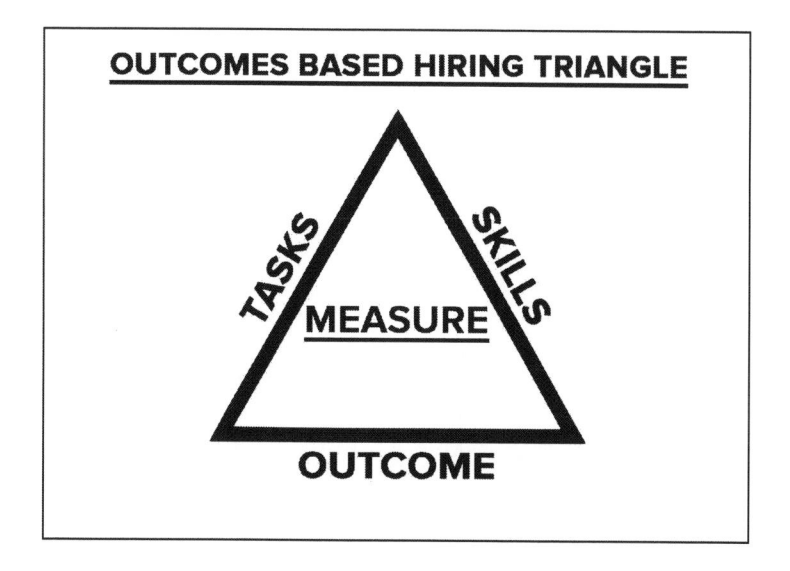

OUTCOMES BASED HIRING TRIANGLE

TASKS / SKILLS / MEASURE / OUTCOME

It is important to understand that, as with any job ad, you are not looking to attract as many people as possible. You only want enough of the *right* people, those with the right capabilities to achieve the outcome you have established. Contrary to popular belief, one of the worst things you can do in the recruitment process is have *too many* people apply for the same role.

Think about it: when you are recruiting you are already overstretched. Time is not your friend, and that is why you are hiring in the first place. When you're "skimming" through 150 resumes, it's highly likely that the one who had the skills you actually need is missed – you didn't pay enough attention because it was at the back of the pile.

Here's what *most* job ads look like:

> **"We have an exciting opportunity for someone who is hard working and committed, who is professional and is reliable, and who has a proven track record of demonstrating results and owning their department. If you're interested, send your CV to…"**

Yawn! Yawn! Yawn!

That type of job ad is not going to help anyone decide whether what you're offering is uniquely suited to them; it is going to have every one think that it is for them. After all, who do you know who doesn't think of themselves as being hard working and committed, or as being professional and reliable?

Let's face it, even the guy or girl who just got fired for being unreliable (for the fifth time) thinks that they were fired unfairly, or that they are yet to find a boss who "understands" them…

When creating any job ad, you need to realize that you're marketing the role in the same way you would when recruiting new patients for your practice. That means attracting the right people and repelling the rest. The sign of a great marketing campaign is one that makes it easy for people to rule themselves in or out, and you must apply the same rules here.

In marketing you're calling out to people who want the things you can achieve for them. Such as; independence, mobility, a lifetime without pills or just being more active. In hiring, you're calling out to people who can achieve the outcomes you are looking for. You are making it very clear that if they don't have the skills to achieve such outcomes, then they should not apply.

This is why you absolutely must complete the *Success Description* before you run any ad to fill a role at your clinic. It is the only way to be clear on what these things actually are.

THE 5 PARTS OF THE JOB AD

Let's look specifically at how to create the ad. With the *Success Description* completed you can now easily pull content from it to create the ad which will attract your perfect candidates.

There are five sections to any job ad that I run:

- **Part 1** - Call out to the person you're looking for
- **Part 2** – Sell the role, you, and your company
- **Part 3** – Explain the responsibilities/tasks they will be doing
- **Part 4** – Skills, Qualifications & Experience required
- **Part 5** – What you will do for the candidate

The image below is the structure of how these parts appear in the ad:

FIG.9

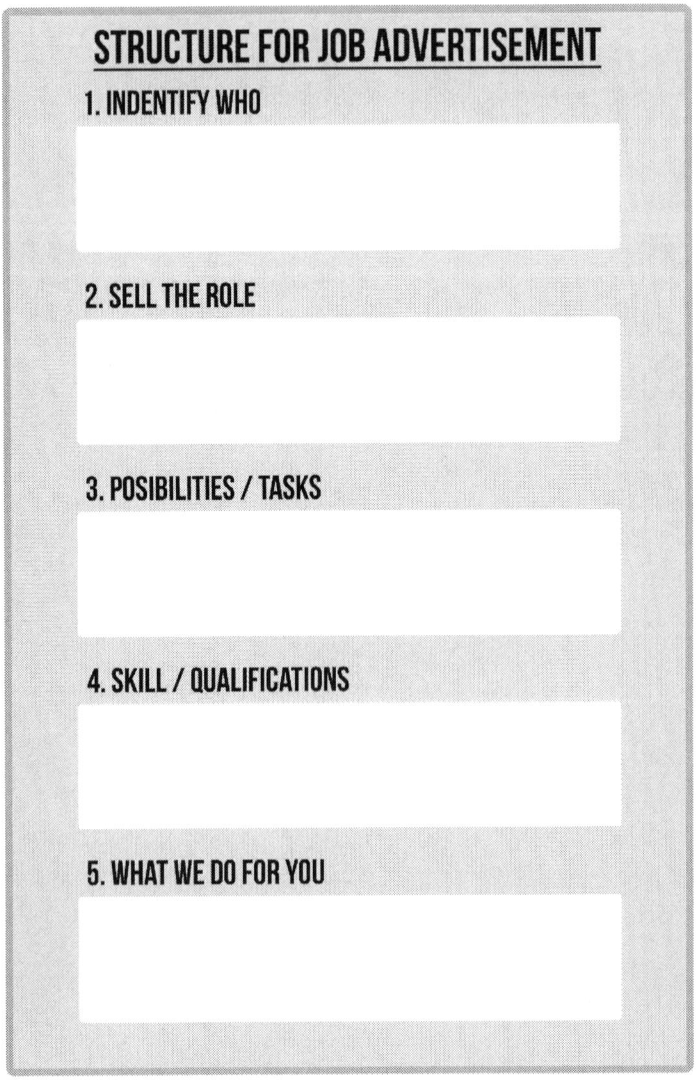

STRUCTURE FOR JOB ADVERTISEMENT

1. INDENTIFY WHO

2. SELL THE ROLE

3. POSIBILITIES / TASKS

4. SKILL / QUALIFICATIONS

5. WHAT WE DO FOR YOU

Tip: if you want to get a real-life example of a recent job ad that I created for a front desk person, be sure to download the resource PDF that accompanies this book. Do that here: **www.paulgough.com/hiring-resource**

PART 1: CALL OUT TO THE PERSON YOU'RE LOOKING FOR

In this first section you're helping people find themselves in the role. This is not about telling them "what they will be responsible for", just like so many ads do; instead, it is telling them what they must possess in order to consider applying, or, even reading the rest of the ad. You need to talk about the things that you're looking for in this person, such as their personal qualities, values, and even their experience in solving the problem that you've got (note: this is very different from experience in your exact role, as the latter is not always needed if you know what skills you require).

WHAT TO SAY IN THE AD FOR THE FRONT DESK/ADMIN PERSON

Here's how it might look for an admin:

> "Are you comfortable with talking to strangers, both in person and on the phone? Are you a self-starter? Is being "organized" a top priority in your life, and are you able to multi-task and prioritize projects while simultaneously meeting deadlines and prioritizing your day?"
>
> "Can you communicate effectively with people from all different backgrounds – both written and verbal? Are you able to speak up when you see something that is not working, and can you anticipate the needs of other people, showing up for work knowing that the smallest details always make the difference?"
>
> "Do you have a positive outlook on life? Are you flexible, open to change, and committed to learning?"

Notice how those things mainly talk about the **type of person** I want. What's more, I am beginning to weed out the people who do not fit the bill for the type of person that I want at my front desk.

If you need to be around someone and be under constant supervision – do not apply. If you can't anticipate the needs of my patients – do not apply. If you are not comfortable with talking to strangers (my patients) on the phone and or in person – do not apply. If you are not committed to learning and you don't like change – **do not apply.**

These are some of the things that I value as a business owner. Any business is a reflection of its owner, and the **values** of the owner. That's why I want to make sure that anyone who applies for one of my jobs has those same values too.

The values you choose dictate most of the problems you inherit in your life. It is the same in a business. There's no point in me telling you what you will be responsible for until we've established shared values. These values will always supersede any other trait or quality that I am looking for, and that's why I get them in early.

I believe that when people talk about "hiring people for personality", what they really mean is, "hire for values"; they just don't articulate it that way. And *that* is what's causing confusion over what employers are looking for.

Personality is very subjective – it can change like the weather. It's people's *values* that you should be considering, as these things rarely ever change. You, as an employer, will certainly never change them. That is why you want to know more about their values than their personality. Specifically, do their values match up to yours? If not, there's likely to be a clash when you ask them to learn new things, embrace change, or go over and above to make people feel special.

WHAT TO SAY IN THE AD FOR A PHYSICAL THERAPIST

Next, here's an example of the type of thing you might say in the job ad for a **physical therapist**:

> "Do you have a positive persona that makes patients look for any excuse to come back and see you? Are you a self-starter? Are you comfortable with picking up the phone to speak to past patients?"
>
> "Are you able to communicate with patients in such a way that they know what you're doing for them? Are you able to connect and engage with people on a personal level (not just clinical skill level)? And, do you have time for people over and above their allocated clinical sessions which you are being paid to give?"
>
> "Do you love to learn, and are you committed to being part of a TEAM that puts the patient first, not professional ego? Are you flexible and open to change? Do you view the opportunity to learn as a privilege and not something that you should be paid to do?"

Again, this ad calls out to the qualities and values that I am looking for in the person fulfilling the role for me. It matters little what those qualities actually are, as long as they are the ones that <u>you</u> want, and the ones <u>you</u> require to be successful at your clinic. If you don't know what your businesses core values are, I strongly suggest you take the time to work them out. It'll save you a lot of heartache when it comes to hiring – and it'll actually make firing easier too.

I do consider personality important. But not before values or skills. Personally, I want someone with the type of personality that my patients are going to, quite literally, "fall in love with". I do not look for people who my patients will "like". I look only for people who my patients will "love" being around.

I am not even remotely interested in their clinical skills –at first. In my humble opinion, the skill aspect of it is not the needle mover as to why people come back and see therapists… it's the therapist's relationship with them.

I want a therapist whose patients will talk about their therapist to everyone that they come into contact with; even someone patients are reminded of when they think about their own sons or daughters. So, my ads call out to those qualities and values.

The job ad goes on to talk about other things that I am going to be expecting of them. For example, I am relentless about in-house training, and I expect my staff to volunteer their time to learning – not just be paid for it. I have an agreement with them: I will compensate them for 50% of the time I allocate in the week for training and development, but they must give up 50% of their time as well.

So, for example, every Wednesday I allocate 3 hours to training. During this time the clinic is closed. My therapists get paid for 1.5 hours; the other hour and a half is their own time. Here's the key point: they do not *have* to show up for the other 1.5 hours if they don't want to. It is not contractually binding and I can't fire or reprimand them if they don't stay. It is a "gentleman's agreement" (verbal) that I have had with them since the beginning of their employment. Guess how many people in my office stay for all three hours?

That is right, <u>all of them</u>. Every week.

Why? Because in the ad I am calling out people who *do* see the value of learning and don't expect to be paid for it. And that's who I attract. You often get what you're looking for in this life; the key is knowing what you're looking for. Start looking for red cars today and you'll notice more of them than any other day. They were always driving past you, you just weren't looking. I am looking for people who want to learn; the ones who don't want to learn, well, they toddle off to work for the system and spend their whole lives kidding themselves that they do want to learn, but only if they get paid.

I once went so far as to suggest that my staff pay **ME** for the time we spend in training together. It's the most impactful thing that anyone can ever do, so to think that people should always expect payment for the privilege blows my mind. Now, when I first said this a few of them thought I was joking, but I was more than half serious, and if the laws of employment weren't so backwards, I'd try to enforce it…

PART 2: SELL YOU, THE ROLE, AND THE COMPANY'S SUCCESS

Once I've written about the person and who I'm looking for, the next thing I am going to do is sell the role to that person. Do not overlook this. Do not take the stance that they should be the only ones having to sell themselves during this process. They are not the only ones with something to gain. You too stand to gain. You stand to gain a person who can help you grow your business; someone who can solve your business problems.

For both of those reasons you must sell yourself to the candidate as they often have more options than you.

If you could ever watch me do a live interview, you'd know exactly when I've found a candidate that I liked; I'll very quickly change my tone, my posture, and I'll start to talk a lot more. I'll talk faster and more energetically about the company, the role, and my own achievements. That's because I'm selling the role to the person. I don't want to lose them to someone who might have sold a worse role, better.

If you've ever watched Shark Tank, one of my favorite TV shows about investment and small business acumen, you'll see they do it on there, too. These guys are multi-millionaires (some billionaires) who you would think could pick anyone they want to invest in. But, that is not how it works. The moment they realize that they want *that* deal, they start selling themselves, trying to outdo the other sharks in the tank. They describe their own qualities and traits, and they make it obvious why they should be picked. You need to do the same in the ad and interview.

Here's an example of how you might sell your company and the role in the job ad:

> "We are a physical therapy clinic, in Hartlepool, that is experiencing rapid growth. We've grown from one member to a team of 20 people; from having 50 patients per week to now having more than 500 come through our doors.
>
> Ask anyone in town and you'll soon discover we have an incredible reputation in the community and have an abundance of great people ready and waiting for you to serve to the best of your ability.
>
> We believe whole-heartedly in education, and provide an immense amount of training, teaching, and coaching. You'll work with a diverse team: as well as hiring people who live locally, we've got people from all parts of the country, thereby giving you the opportunity to form new friendships and connections.
>
> Demand for this role is always high, and we invite you to apply if you feel confident and able to achieve the tasks and responsibilities listed below.
>
> We know that real A Players love to be held accountable for high standards of performance, which means you'll be given your own key objectives and outcomes. When these are consistently met, you'll experience substantial benefits and privileges."

PART 3: THEIR RESPONSIBILITIES AND TASKS

In the third part of the ad you're going to talk about what will be expected of them - their responsibilities and the tasks that you want them to be able to do for you.

Where are you getting this information? That's right, directly from your *Success Description*. You've already written all of these down so you're literally going to copy and paste these across into this part of the ad.

PART 4: SKILLS AND QUALIFICATIONS COME NEXT

Once you've identified who you are looking for, you've sold the role to them and told them what responsibilities/tasks are going to be required by them, the final thing to do is explain what skills, experience, and qualifications you are looking for. These are coming straight from your *Success Description*.

You can, and should, use this section to talk about any specific experience you need them to have. You may want to mention any courses or "preferred" training / qualifications that you're looking for.

Truth be told, on many occasions I've used this section to say something like: "experience in this exact role is **not** required", or a "university degree is **not** required", and I've had an amazing number of good candidates react to those lines.

That's because the biggest frustration of many great candidates is that they can't get an opportunity. No opportunity, no experience. They have the skill, but not the experience. In my humble opinion, in most cases, skills are more important than experience.

Do not confuse what I am saying here: there's a big difference between skills that solve problems, and experience that is time spent.

Sadly, most employers look for "experience", which is years spent in a role, as proof that the person is going to be a great hire. It is what many default to not knowing what else to look for. But, how many years someone has spent in a particular role is not always a great indicator of how great they'll be working for you. There are a significant number of people out there, with a lot of experience that is only acquired because the hassle of firing them was far greater than the hassle caused by their incompetency.

Bottom line, experience is not the holy grail of hiring A Players.

Personally, I look for candidates with skills that may have been used in other roles. I don't need them to have been in my role exactly. I only need them to have solved my problems. Given that all businesses ultimately have the same problems, it is not that difficult to transfer skills, as long as you know which ones you're looking for. Even for a physical therapist, if they're fresh out of school I want to know if they had a job working in a bar and what they did to increase the likelihood of customers coming back. Because that is what I need them to do for me.

For all those reasons, I will often say, "experience not needed", because many times, it really isn't.

PART 5: WHAT YOU WILL DO FOR THE CANDIDATE

I like to finish the ad by explaining what I will do for the candidate; this is another opportunity to sell the role to the right person and motivate them to follow through on the application. I will talk about how I want to support them, to give them a great career opportunity, and about how there is the possibility for growth in the company: pay rises linked to performance and so on.

Don't miss any opportunity to make your role sound more appealing than any of the others that the candidate is applying for. However amazing you think your company is, I guarantee that yours is not the only job they are applying for. Use your ad to make it sound like it is the only one that they should be applying for. Make it sound as though they'd be crazy to not even consider finding out more.

Remember, there's no greater role for you as a business owner than recruiting the right people. Nothing will ever impact your business in the same way that getting the right people will. Your ability to sell the role is directly proportional to how well you can attract, and subsequently recruit, the right candidates.

So, there you have it: how to create your job ad to attract the right candidates. Once you have it, the next thing to do is post it to as many places as possible so that your perfect candidates will be able to see it. That's what we'll do in the next chapter. Turn the page and I'll show you eleven different places where you can insert your ad so that it gets seen…

9

STEP 5/6:
WHERE TO POST YOUR JOB AD
(11 DIFFERENT PLACES)

"I can't find a physical therapist anywhere", or, *"I just can't find good staff to answer the phone"*. are lines I hear regularly from business owners. However, there's a big difference between looking for and having the intent to actually find an employee. And it's the latter that you are going to need if you want to find great people for your business.

If you're reading this thinking that your town is somehow "different", and that great physical therapists and great front of house staff are hard to find, I've got news for you – they're hard to find everywhere. That doesn't mean that they can't be found though, it just means you have to look in more places than one.

Instead of only posting on Craig's List or Indeed, you may need to widen the search.

With that said, let's walk through 11 different ways you can get in front of great candidates. My personal favorite (and yet somewhat controversial) method for attracting great staff is no.11. I wonder if you are brave enough to put it into action...

WHERE TO POST YOUR JOB ADS

As with marketing for new patients, the same rules apply in hiring -- different media will attract different types of candidates. Patients are looking in different places, and so are candidates; don't assume that, just because *you* would use LinkedIn to find a job, everyone else does. That is not the way it works, and that is also why you need an array of different places in which to look for candidates and post your ad.

Broadly speaking, the best candidates may not be actively looking for jobs or wanting to leave their current roles. However, that doesn't mean that they won't want to leave when they hear about your opportunity. It's your job to put that opportunity in front of them and let them decide.

Here are 11 different ways to do it:

#1: YOUR OWN WEBSITE

I'm a huge of fan of always being in the mode of hiring. I'm always willing to speak to potential superstars no matter how happy I am with my current crop of staff. After all, how would I know that what I've got is better than what is out there if I wasn't always actively looking? My staff may have been the best when I hired them, but what if there's someone out there who is even better?

As you can see from the image on the next page, on my website I have a permanent section that is entitled, "We're Hiring". When anyone clicks on the link, they're taken to a page that allows them to show an interest in either an admin or physical therapist position. They can leave me their email address and telephone number, and, as soon as they complete the form, they'll receive an automated email from me telling them what to do next.

FIG.10 – "WE'RE HIRING" ON PAUL GOUGH PHYSIO ROOMS WEBSITE

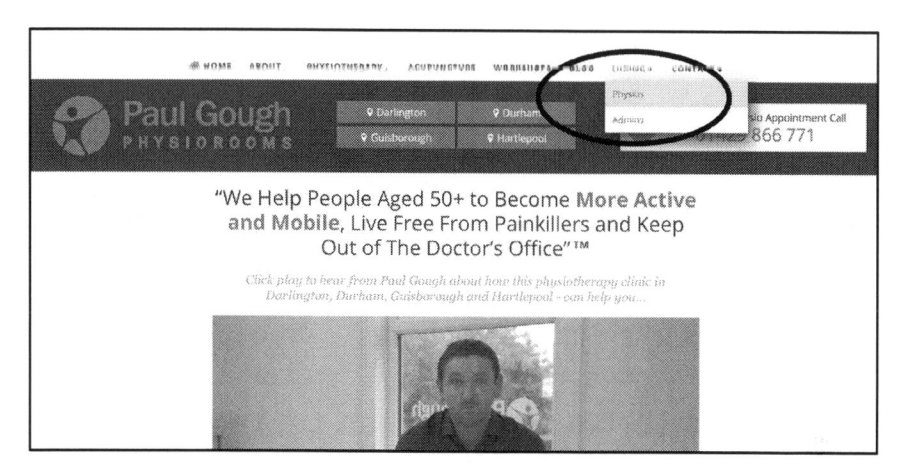

If I am imminently hiring for the role that they have selected, then the instructions will be different from when I am not imminently hiring.

If I'm not hiring any time soon, I will explain in the email that, presently, I do not have a position in need of filling, but that I am always looking to hire superstars. I'll invite the person to make contact with me (by replying to the email), and this paves the way for a very informal chat/interview. We can then talk about what they are looking for and, importantly, begin a relationship with someone who might – just might – be in line for the next role in my office.

Doing this means that I always have a tray full of resumes that I can go to when I next need to hire. It makes it very easy to ring around and see if any of them are still interested in working for me.

#2: YOUR OWN PATIENT LIST

A great place to go to is your own patient list; you should already be communicating with your past patients via email (marketing), so why not use it to advertise the fact that you have a vacant position?

It's really simple to do: in the email (with the subject line: "we're hiring!"), simply announce the fact that an opportunity exists and that you're looking for their help to fill the role. Be very clear on what the role is, who you're looking for, and how they should apply.

You could copy and paste some of the words into the email from your job ad (so that it repels and attracts), and be sure to ask patients, "who do you know?" That is important because the overwhelming majority of them won't be interested, or even skilled, but they'll likely know someone who is.

This is nearly always the very first place I would advertise a role at any time that I am looking to fill a position in any of my businesses. I've even used the *Paul Gough Physio Rooms* email list to fill up roles in *Paul Gough Media*, my marketing business. That's because of the domino effect created, that is, when people tell people, who tell people, and so on.

Sending emails to past patients on a regular basis is often overlooked. I really hope that you're doing it?... Having the ability to email my clients (using Infusionsoft), has not only made hundreds of thousands of dollars, but has also saved tens of thousands of dollars, too. I've been able to fill positions much faster, have not had to pay for ads on traditional job sites, and have attracted quality candidates that come pre-conditioned to want to work for me.

Think about how powerful this strategy is for finding the right people. Any candidate who shows an interest in working for you either knows all about your business already – because they experienced it first hand as a patient – or they've been told all about how cool your company is by a friend who is a patient. Either way, you are getting a very qualified candidate who wants to work for you and doesn't just need a job.

One word of caution on this strategy: every week I have people asking my team if there are any jobs available at my office; *"This seems like a great place to work"* is something we hear all the time. It can be a bit of a problem. Why? Well, because we make it look like such a fun and relaxed place to work. And it is. We *are* very relaxed and we *are* very fun on the outside.

But there's a serious side to everything that we do, too; this is a side that most people do not see. We have outcomes to achieve. That's why, from the get-go, I have to make it very clear that the atmosphere they've experienced happens because of relentless training and focus on making patients our number one priority. The fact that we make it look easy, fun, and a cool place to work is the goal; it is the *effect* of a lot of hard work and training that goes on behind the scenes.

And, one other minor point on this strategy: do not employ the son or daughter of your highest paying patient – just in case you have to fire them! It might cost you in more ways than you bargained for if that situation arises. As of yet, I haven't had to do that, but I did once fire the sister in law of one of my best staff, and another one of her best friends. Oh, and I also fired the wife of a good school friend! *Awkward!*

#3: CONTACT YOUR LOCAL PHYSICAL THERAPY GOVERNING BODY

This is a strategy that is very often overlooked; for most it is never even considered. If you are looking to recruit a physical therapist, then it is highly likely that you'll be able to buy or rent a list of all those qualified in your area from your local/state governing board.

I haven't personally done this, but I've had clients who have been able to buy a mailing list, with the home addresses of hundreds of physical therapists in their area, for less than $100.

When you get the list, all you have to do is write a cover letter explaining the purpose of why you are writing. Then, include the job ad and tell them how to get in touch with you if they want to know more. Refer back to your *Success Description* and write the letter like you would any other ad.

#4: RUN ADS ON FACEBOOK

I've personally had great success with "we're hiring" ads on Facebook, especially for physical therapists and admin staff. This strategy is not to be confused with posting on your personal Facebook or business page. It is about using Facebook's unique ad platform and the incredible targeting power it has.

In my *New Patient Accelerator* marketing book I explained why Facebook is so powerful for finding patients; the social media platform lets you find and display ads that only your perfect patients will see. You can use the same targeting options to find physical therapists in your town – or out of town – or anywhere in the country for that matter.

I've used this strategy with a lot of success; it has helped me get applications from people who were living on the opposite end of the country from my clinic. In fact, here's the exact ad that I used:

FIG.11

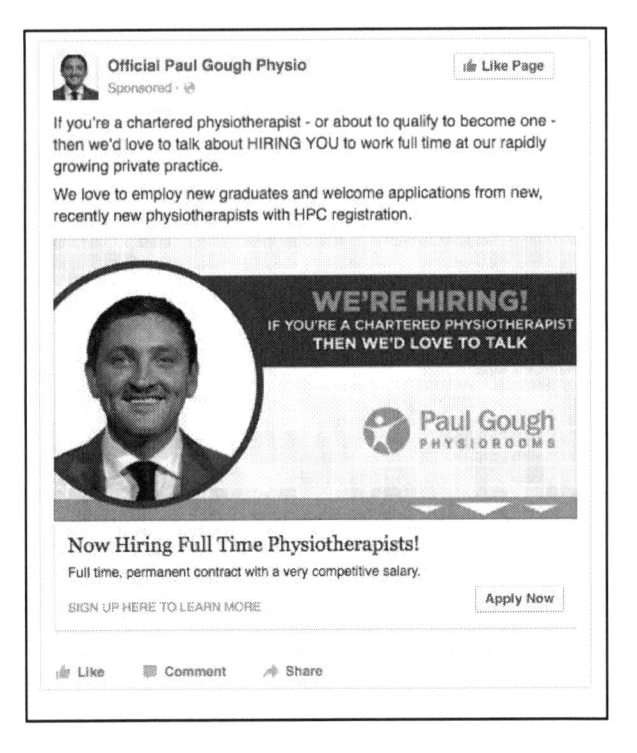

What's more, I've used the same strategy to help a physical therapy clinic in Las Vegas reach physical therapists living across the state line in California, to increase their chances of successfully hiring a superstar.

The same clinic had tried running ads in the local area and all across the usual job sites for months, but with zero response. Using Facebook we were able to target physical therapists from out of state, and we marketed the job so effectively that it compelled people to want to move to another state to take this job.

Note: I've placed a copy of the ad, (and the step-by-step process for making this happen), that we used for this clinic in the resource PDF that accompanies this book. Download it here: **www.paulgough.com/hiring-resource**

Side note: I went into this same clinic in Las Vegas a few months after the person started and I got to meet the girl who got the job from my ad. It was so cool to see the impact of this ad up close. She was very happy in her new job and the company was very happy with their hire! Win-win!

#5: GOOGLE ADWORDS

I use Google Ads to get in front of patients looking for "physical therapy in Hartlepool", and I've used it in the exact same way to get in front of physical therapists looking for jobs in Hartlepool (where one of my clinics is located in the UK).

If you do a quick Google search for the term "physical therapy jobs", you'll likely notice that the top two or three search results are "ads". These ads are paid for by a national company involved in recruitment. Companies run these types of ads in most towns and states, knowing that physical therapists are looking for jobs – everywhere.

When you click, the ad most likely takes you to a website where you can leave your contact details and express an interest in finding out about jobs in the area. And here's the thing: there's nothing stopping you from doing the same.

It's as simple as running an ad on *Google* using the search term "physical therapy jobs in _____ town (just insert your town)". Think about it; the only people searching for that on Google are physical therapists – looking for jobs – in your town! Does it get any easier?

It can cost as little as $10 per day (for two or three weeks) to run an ad and doing that will likely result in a decent number of people looking in that time frame.

Do the math: even if you ran the ad for an entire month it would only cost you $300 to get in front of highly qualified people. These are physical therapists actively searching for a job in your town. There's an argument for permanently running this type of ad to ensure that you're always getting new resumes landing on your desk. Even at $3-$4k per year, it is significantly less than having to pay a recruitment company. You will likely lose a lot more than this if you've got a phone ringing with patients wanting to be seen and no one to schedule them with.

#6: LINKEDIN

You're likely to have the most success on LinkedIn when looking for a physical therapist. For obvious reasons, it's much easier to look for people who are licensed and live in your area on this platform.

Here's a tip: LinkedIn is about building connections. It is about building up a network of contacts. With that said, one of the worst things you can do is go straight to LinkedIn and post that you're looking to hire someone. Sure, it might work. But, what will work better is if you start to build your relationships and connections before you need to hire.

It's so easy for people to abuse these social sites for personal gain. The problem is, when you do that the people who are on LinkedIn every day, don't take to it too well. They're going to be less likely to help you.

If you do as LinkedIn wants, and you build up your connections with the right people over a period of time, what you'll find is that those people will be much more likely to help you. They'll happily share your posts or go out of their way to personally tell someone they know about you and your offers. As I said in the *"How To Create Your Hiring Plan"* chapter, (chapter 5), the more time you have, and the more thought and consideration you give to hiring, the easier it is to be successful at it.

There are likely tens of thousands of people trying to use LinkedIn to find someone to fill a role at this moment – and that's why it won't work for them. Use LinkedIn for its core purpose - connections and relationships, – and you'll fill your roles as a happy by-product.

#7: INDEED/CRAIGSLIST

Most people know about Craig's List and Indeed (and there are many other sites just like those). The only downside to these types of websites is that you will undoubtedly attract a lot of candidates.

Some, if not most, will be completely unqualified/unskilled, and that is why you need to have a process in place that protects you from being inundated with resumes. As I said before, the last thing you want is 150 resumes landing on your desk on the same day.

That said, to get to the best candidates, you need options and choices. These types of sites are still very much worth your time. Just make sure to protect your time by creating an ad that repels and attracts. What's more, later on in the book (Chapter 12), I'll be sharing with you my process for automating the entire hiring process; that invented primarily because of the overwhelming number of resumes I'd get from these types of job sites.

Before I move on, I want to point out again that, although these types of sites should be used, they should not be the *only* ones you use. If this is the only place you post, you really will limit your options for finding quality candidates.

#8: RECRUITMENT AGENCIES

Another obvious place to look for candidates is recruitment agencies. However, and for full disclosure, personally speaking I always try to avoid using these companies at all costs.

Firstly, the cost/risk is a problem; it is so expensive to hire staff through these places.

For a small business owner to take the *risk* on a candidate that could cost you somewhere in the region of 15-20% of their annual salary, you're going to have to be 100% certain. And that simply isn't possible with hiring.

At best, we might be able to tip the odds in our favor from "50-50" to "80-20", but it's never going to work out perfectly every time. Even with the best recruitment process, executed perfectly, there are still so many variables that you cannot control, including illness, change of circumstances in their home, spousal or partner unemployment, or unexpected upheavals.

I've had that exact thing happen to me more than once, so you could say that I am a little "battle scarred"; on two occasions I paid my money to an agency in order to get a great candidate, yet my hire left within just a couple of weeks of the money hitting the agency's account.

One of the candidates was a completely incorrect fit (this happened before I had a proper process like this), and the other left because of a change in her husband's circumstances. She was a great candidate who <u>would</u> have done a great job for us. She also cost me close to $10,000.

Despite all of that, I am not saying do not use an agency. What I am saying, however, is that you should be aware of the risks. The purpose of all my books and teachings is to share with you the lessons I've learned and the mistakes I've made.

As a teacher, I try to "de-risk" the decisions that my students make about their business, and I believe that if you commit to making fewer big/stupid mistakes, you'll be a lot better off.

This is one of those situations. I am sharing a painful lesson with you so that you can make a better judgment regarding whether or not these companies would be right for you. You've got to know that the downside is pretty severe, since there is a lot you cannot control. That's why all of the chapters in this book are important; in particular, understanding the common *hiring mistakes* and *creating a hiring plan* (that you may be tempted to skip).

What you could do, and what I would recommend you do, is use the agencies to compare candidates from other sources. Which means you do not have to hire anyone from these agencies, and also that doesn't mean you can't interview.

Again, I've done this many times over. I've put the role out to the agencies and let them send me candidates who I've then interviewed. On nearly all occasions the stronger candidates actually came from my other recruitment sources (described in this chapter). There is always value in doing this; it allowed me to be more certain and more confident in the person I was hiring, simply because I had seen others.

You wouldn't pick the first house you went to see. To make sure you've really got the house you want, you go to see four or five others first. You should do the same with hiring.

If the one you want is from the agency, then you have a large problem; in this instance, refer back to the "decision framework" (that I taught you in chapter 5). It will all come down to whether or not you can live with the downside of the decision - the $10,000 you might lose to the agency if the candidate walks out after 2 months.

As you grow, you should always have one eye on protecting the downside – it'll get you a lot further in business than constantly chasing a large chunk of the upside. Risk it sometimes, but do so with caution.

#9: SOCIAL MEDIA

The key to using your social media channels (Facebook, Instagram, YouTube, etc.) is to ensure that your post goes *way beyond* just your own network. Sounds elementary, but you want to have everyone you know share the opportunity across their social networks, as well. This includes your current staff.

After all, "birds of a feather flock together." Chances are that your staff are connected to the type of people you want to reach, and it is especially true in the physical therapy community! I've always asked my staff to get involved in posting jobs for me and they have never had a problem with doing it. Why would they? If they were fully committed to helping and supporting the business (that pays their wages), why would they *not* want to do it?

As well as employees, ask everyone from your friends and family, and even patients, to "share this." I once asked my sister to share a job posting that caught the eye of one of her friends, someone who I later hired.

The girl in question wasn't actively looking for a role. However, she wasn't overly happy in the role she was in. You could say that she was waiting for an opportunity to fall into her lap. On this occasion, it fell into her newsfeed on Facebook. This method really can work.

The only problem with this method is that it is neither predictable nor repeatable; you are quite literally "scatter posting" the position to anyone and everyone, which is far from ideal. To make sure that you don't get inundated with too many resumes that are not appropriate, include a little hurdle for them to jump through so that you can separate their intention via inciting action.

For example, you might ask the candidates to include both a resume and a one-page cover letter explaining why they think they are perfect for the job. You'll be amazed at how asking them to do something simple like this puts off the wrong applicants, and in doing so, brings you closer to the right ones.

As an aside, one of the other reasons I like using social media to advertise a role is that it sends positive vibes to your patients; if you position the hiring as "we're growing so fast we need more great people to serve our great patients", it sends positive vibes to your customer base that you're growing, you're successful, and that you're sailing a good ship! People want to be associated with successful companies – patients and staff!

So, don't overlook this method; leverage the additional marketing exposure it can bring you, but make sure you add an extra step like making them write a 500-word cover letter selling themselves on the role.

#10: CONTACT THE LOCAL PT SCHOOLS

One other way you could get in front of physical therapists is to strike up a relationship with the local PT Schools or colleges near you. This could be a long play, but it could also be hugely effective. If you're able to get friendly with, or close to, the relevant people at the school, they'll help you out. That could include posting your vacancy on the notice boards on campus, sending out emails, or just making a bee-line for the top students who are about to qualify to tell them that you're hiring.

I've done this for years, and not just at the university I went to, but at those within a 100-mile radius of my clinic.

I've yet to meet a lecturer or director who doesn't want to help his or her students get a good job. If you spend some time establishing a relationship beforehand, you'll find that you can call them directly and just ask them to post your job; they'll often go one step further for you and go directly to the top five or six students that are about to graduate.

Whether you have a relationship or you don't, this is one of those strategies that you can, and should, just deploy today. Ideally, you do have a pre-existing relationship, but even in the absence of it I am pretty sure that the closest schools would be willing to help you out. Even a month or three after graduation, I've had lecturers personally ring their best students for me to see if they're still looking for a job.

If they help you out, be sure to help them out. Promise a guest lecture, or you take one of their students on as a placement in the next year or so. One good turn deserves another.

#11: PERSONALLY WRITE TO ALL THE CLINICIANS IN TOWN — AT THEIR CURRENT PLACE OF WORK (GASP!)

This is the one that some people reading the book might find a little controversial, but what the heck! All is fair in love and war.

Besides, I learned about this strategy the hard way and I've come to acknowledge that it was, and is, a great strategy that cuts out time and puts you straight in front of the people you want.

I can still remember the day it happened to me; I was looking at the mail one day and wondering why every single member of my staff *all* had a letter that day, all written in the same handwriting, in the same envelope, and from the same sender. I was on the receiving end of a clinic in my town trying to poach my staff! They took it upon themselves to write to all of my staff members and ask if they wanted new jobs!

Yes, this clinic, which was a competitor of mine, wrote to every one of my staff and basically asked them if they wanted a pay rise!

What a brilliant way to solve your problem!

This clinic had simply gone onto my website and looked for the names of all my therapists – and then wrote to each one at my main clinic. Neither is that difficult to do.

As you can imagine, at first I was a little angry. But, then I changed my view of what they had done; it was genius: a "renegade" way of solving a problem in their business. I just happened to be on the receiving end of it. That doesn't change how good of an idea it was.

When you stop and think about it, this is probably the best of all of the strategies you could deploy. You're going straight to the heart of it. You're directly targeting the people in jobs that you need filling in your own business.

I guarantee you it works, too. How do I know? Because I lost one of my staff members in the process… one who took a $6k pay rise! Send a letter to 10 people in any company asking, "are you happy in your role – and if not, would you like to talk about how my role might be a good fit?", and you *will* get at least one who replies.

It is statistically not possible for everyone who gets a "are you happy?" letter, to actually be happy.
Sure, they may not all be looking for a new job, but heads are turned when they get a letter like this.

I fully endorse this strategy, and having been on the receiving end of it, I'm in a comfortable position to say so. I have no problems at all with doing it or having it done to me again. That's because, if one of my staff members does want to leave, they've likely saved me a lot of hassle; the hassle that comes with carrying an underperforming staff member who had (or is about to) loose interest in my company.

Had my staff member not taken the job, it wouldn't have been too long before that same person would have sucked oxygen from my business – hanging around for months while looking for a new job. If I had ever met the owner of the clinic who did it, I would have thanked him or her.

Here's another thing to understand; if more than one person is leaving, then I have found a new problem in my business: my leadership! That's right. I'd be thankful of someone doing it again, resulting in a mass exodus, as it would be exposing the real problem in my business – "me".

The other clinic in town sending letters is not the issue, and staff leaving after having responded to the letters is not the issue either. That is the **effect**. My poor culture and leadership is the **cause**, and once I know it's an issue, I can set about fixing it.

So, if you're planning on doing it to me, I say *thank you* in advance. And, the address of my clinic is proudly displayed on my website…

If you're thinking of doing this, but you're worried that the other clinic owner might not like you, guess what? They probably don't like you anyway.

To do this, first up you will need a little bit of "balls". When/if you've found them, just head over to the websites of all of the clinics in your area and find the names of the staff in the staff section. Be sure to do it to all the clinics – I don't want you being accused of discriminating against anyone.

If you can't find the names listed on the website then that's not a problem either; just call up the secretary and ask something like this: "I'm interested in booking an appointment at your clinic, and so that I can check their registration meets my insurance, <u>can I please have the full names of all your therapists?</u>"

I guarantee that they will give them to you. How do I know? I've done it many, many times.

When you mail them, don't be disrespectful to their employer. Just simply write a letter asking, "are you happy in your current role?", and suggest that if they're not (happy), "would you like to talk about an opportunity I have that might make you a little happier – and perhaps even richer?"

With that type of wording, your phone will be ringing off the hook.

Try it, I am very sure it'll solve your recruitment issues, and this would be the first thing that I would do if was in urgent need of hiring a physical therapist.

So, there you have it. 11 different strategies to get your job opportunity in front of the right candidates. It really is amazing how simple it is to find people – as long as you look in the right places and commit to building the right relationships.

The worst mistake is to conclude that, just because you placed an ad on Indeed, and because no one responded, that "there's no one out there".

If you're serious about hiring great people, you'll use at least 6 or 7 different methods at the same time. You'll soon discover that there are good people out there waiting to be hired. You just had to go a little further than Craig's List or a sign in your clinic window to reach them.

Ok, so far we have been recruiting - next, let's move into the actual hiring phase. We'll look at the interview process and specifically, what questions to ask.

10

STEP 6/6:
THE INTERVIEW PROCESS
(AND WHAT QUESTIONS TO ASK)

Over the last few chapters we've come a long way. We've *created a plan for hiring*, considered what the *financial metric of success* looks like, created a *Success Description* – and all from that, we've pulled a *job ad* that we can post in at least *11 different places*. Now with the ad working, candidates are starting to respond, and it's time to move from the recruitment phase to the hiring phase.

In this chapter we're going to walk through the 6-part interview process that I've used to hire A Players - the type of candidate that every business owner dreams of.

This entire model for hiring has been a work in progress for close to ten years; meaning, I've optimized this process over the years to get it to where it is today. I use 6 steps that will first <u>eliminate</u> all of the B and C Players, leaving me with a 'crop" of potential A Players from which to find the one superstar that I want to hire.

Here's a quick re-cap of the two main objectives that should guide you at this point:

- **Interviews** – provide the facts you need in order to rate a person against the *Success Description* you have created for the role.

- **A Players** – those who have a track record that matches your needs and have the skills that will align with your culture and your role.

What's more, the true, widely accepted definition of an A Player is someone who is in the top 15% of their pay bracket.

So, for example, someone in the top 15% of a $25,000 salary bracket is classed as an A Player. What that also means is if the same person moved up and into a $30,000 bracket, they might not be considered an A Player. This is important to understand – it forces you to think objectively about who it is you're hiring. Just because they interview well, or present with a great track record, it doesn't mean that you've automatically found an A Player.

This also means that it is possible that the A Player you're looking for can be found in the pay bracket below the one you think you need to advertise for; that someone in the upper end of the $20-25k bracket is better than someone in the lower end of the $25-30k bracket.

To that end, something that I've not been afraid to do over the years is run similar job ads, for the same role advertised, but with different salaries. That's because people usually look for jobs according to what they think they are worth. Most candidates have an idea of the salary bracket that they *think* they're in and will therefore apply for jobs within that range.

It doesn't mean they are worth that amount; it just means that is what they think they are worth. When you do this, you'll be surprised to learn that advertising a higher salary does not always attract the best candidates. Sometimes it does, but not always.

The point I am raising? There's more than one way to achieve the outcome you want. Don't get stuck on thinking that an A Player is going to cost you the earth. They're not. Just make sure you select someone in the top 15% of the bracket that you're advertising for.

Now you know what an A Player really is, let's look at the 6-steps in this interview process:

1. The initial phone interview (screening to rule out B and C Players).

2. The first in-person interview (focus on personality, values, previous track record).

3. The second in-person interview (focused on primary objective of the role).

4. Meet the team.

5. Check references.

6. Make the offer (and potentially negotiate).

PART 1: THE INITIAL PHONE INTERVIEW (GOAL: RULE OUT B AND C PLAYERS)

At the beginning of the hiring process I am simply looking to rule out the candidates who have applied for the wrong job. I'm looking to narrow down my candidate pool, from the 20 or so, to the 7 or 8 who are qualified and able to fulfill the role. There is a difference.

I do this by "screening" the initial candidates on the phone. Whether I am looking for a physical therapist, a front of house/admin, an operations manager for my marketing company, or a financial controller, I always start by narrowing down the pool of candidates to ones that are obviously more suitable.

Key point: I do not do this part. I will ask someone in my office to do it for me. I'll ask one of my front desk people to do it for me, as it really is about *getting a feel* for who the person is and what they're looking for. What's more, trying to get 20 people on the phone is a mammoth task in and of itself!

The time it takes getting hold of all these candidates is often underestimated, as you're often playing phone tag with people who could be great candidates. I trust the judgment of my staff implicitly, and this is their chance to take part in the development and progress of the clinic. However, you must not relinquish complete control: give the staff member an objective (find the best 7 or 8), give them a time frame in which to do it (i.e. 7 days), and give instructions for *what questions to ask*.

This whole phase is about finding out if the person who applied for your role and their career goals, match up to what you can provide them.

You're also looking for how they say what they say. How did they handle the conversation with your team? Are they bright and bubbly? Are there any awkward silences? Do they answer with a yes or no? Or, can they develop and lead a conversation? Do they talk too much? Do they talk in a way that will send you to sleep? Is there any enthusiasm for this particular role and working for your company?...

...Or, do they just want a job and a salary? These are all of the things you are looking for; this part allows you to build a profile of the person, therefore slowing you to decide if they should advance to the next phase.

Some questions you **might** ask, include:

Q. What are your career goals?

You are listening for the candidate's goals and passions – and you want those passions to be aligned with the role.

Q. What are you really good at, professionally?

You are looking for 8 or 12 positive attributes to build a complete picture of their professional capability. Ask for examples to put their strengths into context. If they say they are "decisive", ask for examples of when they were decisive, and so on!

Q. What are you not good at or not interested in doing, professionally?

You may probe and say, "what would your reference say about what you are not good at or not interested in?"

Q. Who were your last 5 bosses, and how will they rate your performance on a scale of 1-10 <u>when</u> we talk to them?

The key word here is "when" I call them. Do not say "if" I called them. The use of *when* implies that you will be calling them, and therefore candidates are more likely to tell the truth…

Q. What specifically have you done in the field of _____X_____

Insert the #1 one problem you are solving… if it is a retention issue, ask them about retaining customers. If it is an acquisition issue, talk to them about how they've acquired customers before.

My experience is that this phase really isn't all that difficult. The hardest part is getting them on the phone in the first place, and this is why you should consider someone else doing it for you. The objective is to simply separate the good from the bad (and the ugly). Don't obsess over it – just literally move forward with what your first instinct is on the candidate. The potential A Players will stand out in the way can answer these questions; <u>it's mostly about how they say it,</u> not necessarily what they say.

If in doubt, put them through to the next step. Follow my whole process and it has enough traps built into it so that you'll catch the bad ones eventually. As you move on to the next part of the interview, you can probe a lot more with your questions, taking more time to consider their answers.

PART 2: THE FIRST IN PERSON INTERVIEW

At this point, you're hopefully down from a group of 20 initial candidates, to a smaller pool of 7 or 8 with real potential to contain the one you want. Now, this is where you'll go deeper into questions about their previous roles and what they've done for other people – as well as discovering more about their personalities and their values.

Both of these are equally as important as the other. Ideally, I'm hoping to find someone whose values align to the ones I've set for the business – and who is skilled enough to solve my problems.

Back to what I said in the earlier chapters of this book: it is not enough to hire <u>solely</u> on values and personality. This process is about, firstly, finding people with the right values (often confused as personality), and secondly, picking the best one based on their skill level and ability to solve your problems.

To get into that position, you have to ask the right questions - questions that will give you clues about what they've done for other employers, the likes of which will correspond to what you will need them to do for you.

The ideal position to be in is a strong pool of candidates who have some history of solving a problem that is in some way similar to the one you have.

For example, if it is a lead conversion role, candidates can vividly tell you about many situations involving prospects that they have spoken with that have ended with money being handed over.

And if it is a physical therapist, have they got some experience of what it takes to get customers to come back to a business... even if it is waiting tables at a restaurant during college!

It is important to talk more about what they <u>have done</u>, rather than asking what they *might* do. That is a big distinction to make.

Resist asking them about situations in the future that have not even happened. Asking them, "how might you deal with this situation....", is doing nothing but testing their imagination. They are not being paid to imagine; they are being paid to solve problems that will lead to a more profitable business. You should only ever be asking questions about **how** they have dealt with situations. This is going to give you facts. Facts are always better than theory.

HOW TO START THE INTERVIEW

When the interview starts, I am rarely in the room. That is because I am nearly always five minutes (or so) late when I do my interview – on purpose.

At my place, the interview starts from the moment they enter the clinic, interacting with the other staff and even the patients who are waiting in reception. I want to see how the person talks to the other people in my clinic while they're waiting for me.

How they interact with others in my office is something else that I can note down as I build the profile. After the interview is over, I'll go and talk to the staff in order to get their opinion about how the candidates conducted themselves when they first walked in.

I always start the first interview by talking for 3-5 minutes. I ensure that the candidates understand the full nature of the role they are applying for. I'll then explain that this is a 30-minute interview with the view of cutting down the field to a list of no more than 3 or 4.

I find if you talk for a few minutes first, it also allows the candidate to get more comfortable with you. Which is important. Remember that they're nervous, and this person could potentially solve a huge problem for you. That's why you should do everything you can to create the optimal environment; one that'll give them the opportunity to be the best version of themselves.

Interestingly, most of the best employees I've ever hired didn't start well – but, they came into their own once they got their confidence and started enjoying the process. It is in your best interests to create that type environment.

DISCOVERING THEIR VALUES - AND MATCHING THEM TO YOURS

I touched on this earlier in the book: to have any chance of being successful in your hiring you absolutely must be looking for people who have the same values as you have established. It's more important to consider the persons values than it is to have an opinion on their personality.

Discovering your clinics **core values** is such an important process. In fact, it's so fundamental that in my "Physical Therapy Business Growth School" program, (6-week online virtual training), I devote an entire module to helping owners establish and live by those values.

Having the right values not only allows you to run your clinic according to those values, it also allows you to hire and fire according to them. It is how you're confidently able to leave the clinic knowing that others know how to handle things in your absence. You show me a clinic owner who can't leave their clinic and I'll show you one who is devoid of values that staff were hired for.

Once you know what your values are, you can start asking one or two questions with those values acting as your guide. This is to see if you and the person you're talking to are a match.

For example, one of the core values at my clinic is "pursue growth and learning". The happiest people are learning. They are growing all the time. I only want to be around people who are growing and learning, because I am constantly doing both. If I am ever around people who are not growing and learning, two things happen: I irritate them and they irritate me. That's why I would never employ anyone who doesn't love to learn.

However, it is one thing for someone to tell you they like to learn, but it is another thing for them to demonstrate it. That is why I might ask a question like this:

Q. "Tell me about the last three things you've learned – that were not paid for by someone else, or that didn't include the required Con. Ed or CEU courses which are mandatory to maintain your license. What were they and why did you choose them?"

After asking that question, one of two things will happen:

1. There'll be a stunned silence (not good!).

2. The candidate will tell you about how they've invested in online training programs, books, attended a personal growth seminar, or just bought a DVD program that is about how to be better at something.

What I am looking for here is not *what* they did or *why* they did it – only the fact that they did it. Anyone can, and will, **say** that they value learning if you ask them in an interview situation. But, if they have no history of doing it (except what is necessary to keep their PT license), then they simply don't value learning. What they are saying is that they would like to value learning, but just not enough to actually sacrifice something and pay for it.

Another core value that I have at my clinic is this: "anticipate the unspoken needs of the patient". To find out if the person I am talking to values that as well, I might ask something like:

Q. "Tell me about a time when you were able to anticipate an unspoken need of a customer. What was the situation and how did it end?"

It may take them a few seconds (that's ok, they're just recalling information – so let them think!), but this is going to test their ability to recognize when they've done such a thing and how they were able to execute it. Again, you're not really concerned with what it was, only that they did it and could recognize it.

Another one of my 10 core business values is, "create WOW factor experiences". So, with that in mind, I am going to be asking about their previous roles with the intention of hearing about times when they went over and above to create a memorable, WOW factor experience. The question might be:

Q. "Tell me about a time in a previous role when you turned a routine situation into something that made the customers happy or smile unexpectedly?"

Again, I am not concerned with what it was, only that they have done it.

The phrase, "don't tell me you love me – show me you love me", sums this up perfectly. All of your questions must be look for proof that they've done what you're asking.

This is the part of the interview where the personality thing is considered; only, I am not looking at their personalities, I am looking at what they value. Focus on their values and matching them up to yours, and you'll find that people are happy to bring their personalities to your work.

Said differently, they can have the happiest personality on earth, but that personality is going to quickly change the moment your values clash! When you have opposing values it is almost impossible for any relationship to survive.

Really, it should be "hire for values", not "hire for personality".

QUESTIONS THAT REVEAL THEIR SKILL LEVELS

With the value questions covered, the next thing I'm asking for is proof of a skill set or competencies demonstrated in their previous role.

I want to know about what they've done in the past, and I want to see if I can match that up to what I know I will need them to do for me. I am going to talk about what they've previously been hired to do in-depth. I'll ask the candidate to pick a job (ideally one that matches the one they are applying for), and then begin asking a series of questions about that role so I can continue to build a profile from their answers.

Here are some examples of questions that I might ask:

Q. What were you hired to do?

I am asking this question to find out if the person had a deep understanding of the real reason they were hired. For example, they might say, "to answer the phone to customers". But, that isn't why they were really hired. Sure, that might have been one of their tasks, but it is unlikely why they were hired.

I am ideally looking for answers like, "I was hired to provide customers with enough information to make confident purchase decisions and ensure that the same customer returns to us time and time again". Now *that* is how a superstar answers the question of what they were hired to do.

Q. What accomplishments are you most proud of?

By talking about successes that they've had in the past, they're going to get comfortable very early on. Hopefully, the candidate will be able to recall things that they're proud of and, by happy coincidence, you'll listen for if/how those accomplishments are relevant to the things that you'll need this person to do for you in your job opportunity.

Q. What were some low points during that job?

When I ask this question, I am looking to see if the candidate is able to recognize when things are not going so well – and be ok with talking about it. The last thing I want is to hire an eternal optimist who thinks that everything is permanently rosy. Business does not work like that, and I would much rather have someone on my team who can tell me how it is, not how they wish it would be.

You may want to probe when they answer this question, asking one or two more questions about how they played a part in resolving the issue and how it ended. It's not a deal breaker of a question in any way. Far from it, actually; you're just building a rounded profile and hoping to find clues about their performance/behavior that are real and not canned interview responses.

Q. Who were the people you worked with? Specifically: What was your boss's name and how do you spell that? What was it like working with him/her? What will they tell me about your biggest strengths and areas for improvement?

This question sends a message to the candidate that *I am* going to be checking up on what their previous boss would say. It means that they are much more likely to tell me the truth in the interview. I am looking for how they talk about their boss; are they respectful? Do they blame everyone they work with for their failures or frustrations?

Do they say that they couldn't get along with their boss? Or, are they honest and rounded in their explanation of the relationship? All of these things give me clues as to who this person really is and how they see their boss. I guarantee that however they see their current boss is most likely how they will *eventually* see you...

Q. How would you rate the performance of the department you were hired in? What changes did you make? How would you rate the department that you left on a scale of A, B, C?

What this tells me is whether or not the person had any impact on the business since they were employed. Did they make a difference? If they doesn't think they made any difference, then I'm not sure I want him or her working for me.

Now, they might tell me that they tried to do a lot of things that were blocked by someone in a higher position, and that is ultimately why they're leaving. If they answer in this way, I'll probe with more questions about their reasons for wanting to make the changes. What problems did they see? What solutions were they offering? All of this is going to help me understand their judgments and desires for wanting to succeed in my job.

In the final question of this part of the interview, I make it very specific to a problem that I want solved or the outcome I expect from them.

For example, **if I was hiring a physical therapist**, one of the things that I deemed crucial when creating my *Success Description* is being able to have patients complete a recommended plan of care.

Therefore, I would ask something like this:

Q. "What, specifically, have you achieved in the field of retaining your patients? And, what is the extent of your understanding about what it takes to ensure that a patient completes a full plan of care?"

Expect there to be a little silence when you ask this type of question… for two good reasons:

1. You judge a great question by the length of the silence after you ask it (the longer, the better).
2. They've never heard a question like this before, so it will take a few seconds to process (no other boss they've worked

for would ever think of asking questions related to outcomes.)

The answer is going to give you a greater understanding of the candidate, specifically where this person <u>currently is</u> with regards to one of the crucial things you have deemed important for success in the role. I am not hiring them solely on this answer, but I *am* making a judgment on how big their knowledge gap is in this area – I am making a note of how much training is required from me if I hire them.

THE BEST ONES MUST DO A HOMEWORK TASK

If I deem the candidate a good fit, and I want them to advance in the interview process, I'll always ask them to do a task in between this interview and the next one (the focused interview).

I do this for a couple of reasons. The first reason is to put up another barrier for anyone who is trying to breeze their way into my role. There are lots of "professional interviewees" lurking out there – people who can say the right things and look the right way – but, it doesn't mean they'll become great employees. Asking people to do a task that is going to cost them their *time* is one way of weeding these people out.

Secondly, I always get to learn something; the task that I set is always related to the role I need filling, and by asking candidates to do a presentation, or to prepare something related to their role, they nearly always bring something to my attention that I had not thought of. Doing *this* means I really look forward to the interview process for more reasons than just finding a quality candidate to solve problems in my business.

Thirdly, asking them to do a task also allows you to see what the candidate is like in a way that is difficult to create in your typical interview environment.

If they are preparing presentations, you'll get to notice things like confidence, communication skills, attention to detail, and ability to improvise when you ask an off-the-cuff question. Not to mention simple things like their punctuation, grammar, and spelling. If you ask three candidates to do the same task, you'll really get a feel for what the difference is between them all.

Where are their strengths and weaknesses? And, is what they have told you consistent with what you've seen so far?

Again, none of this is *getting* them the job or *not getting* them the job – it is letting you build the case for hiring the right one.

During the interview process it is important to understand that no one single answer, question, attribute, demonstration of skill, or other benefit is going to get them the job. Much like a lawyer building a case against a criminal in a courtroom, there's no one single piece of evidence powerful enough to convict the criminal. It is the compound effect of all the pieces of evidence that is going to add up to whether or not the jury will convict.

If the prosecution relies on just one strong piece of evidence, they won't be that confident about the decision no matter how well the glove fits! Same with hiring: if you're choosing a candidate based on one stand out feature or thing that you like, you *may* get the decision right, but it's risky. You'll find yourself sweating over the decision for quite some time after you've hired them. My tip is to look at all of these phases as allowing you to build your candidate profile. This includes the task they must complete for you.

WHAT TYPE OF HOMEWORK TASK MIGHT YOU HAVE THEM DO?

So, what do you ask them to do? Well, in the case of a **physical therapist**, I know that one of the things I want them to be doing for me is to ensure a completed plan of care ratio above 90%. With that in mind, I could ask them to prepare a presentation – as though they were teaching my other staff – about the top 6 things needed for a patient to complete a plan of care.

This does two things:

Firstly, it is in line with the values of my business, ones we have hopefully already agreed that we share – a love of learning. By asking the candidate to prepare a presentation on the topic of retention, I am about to find out if they are prepared to spend a couple of hours of their own time studying.

Secondly, I am about to discover their true understanding of a vital part of the role they are applying for. It is the perfect scenario.

In the case of a **front of house/front desk** role, an example of a homework task that you might ask them to do is to prepare a presentation; ask them to explain the difference between a physical therapist and a chiropractor. Or, ask them to outline the true benefits of physical therapy as they might explain it to a patient.

What matters is not so much what they say at this point, but rather that they are willing to do it. And, furthermore, that they take the time to research two points which are, essentially, two very common questions that they will be asked when patients call up to book appointments.

Don't obsess too much over the task, just try to have them take part in something that will give you an insight into who they really are. Ideally, it is in some way linked to one of the major outcomes they'll be held accountable for when working for you.

That's part 2 concluded. The goal is to invite the shortlist back for a second interview and then focus on one or two specific aspects of the role.

Let's look at how to do it…

PART 3: THE SECOND IN-PERSON INTERVIEW

If the candidate has made it this far, it's because they've shown that they own values similar to those that are important for my business.

They've also demonstrated some level of competency or displayed skills that I am looking for in a previous role. Now, in this second interview (that usually takes place a week later), I want to go deeper.

This phase is where I am going to narrow in on one or two specific topics; they are key to the success of the role, and I'll ask a lot of questions within those specific one or two topics.

I am going to "probe" deeper into any answers they give me, and I'm looking for clues – insights – about their real understanding and skill level in these particular areas. I've heard this phase of the interview process called the "focused" interview, and that's exactly what it is; you're focusing on the one or two things that, if they just accomplished these for you, would make this hire a success.

SPECIFIC QUESTIONS ABOUT THE SPECIFIC OUTCOMES YOU NEED

So, let's look at some specific questions that you might ask in this phase - we'll start with a physical therapist. Remember, all of my questions being asked here are because I consider the most important aspect of their role to be retention.

You might consider it something else – and that's fine – just copy my thinking and follow the framework for how you decide which questions to ask. What matters most is that you're aware of the outcome that you want for this person. If you have that, then you're able to switch-up the questions in order to give you insights into how capable this candidate is at achieving *that* outcome. That is what the questions do.

Here are some examples of questions that I might ask in the interview:

Q1. The purpose of this interview is to talk specifically about your ability to keep patients on schedule:

   a. What are your biggest accomplishments in this area during your career?

   b. What is your current understanding of why patients "drop off", or cancel, mid-way through a plan of care, and what can be done to mitigate those factors?

   c. What are your biggest mistakes and lessons learned in this area?

   d. Tell me about a time in the past where you've had to deal with a patient who had a high copay or huge excess, and who was reluctant to pay (even though they needed treatment). How did you handle the situation, and what did you do to ensure it ended successfully for both of you?

   e. Based on your current role, what ideas do you have that could improve the *completed plan of care* rate at your current clinic?

The second area that I would want to probe regarding a physical therapist would be their ability to handle patient objections - objections or push back about booking sessions.

With the cost of health care rising, you're seeing more and more patients reluctant to complete the plan of care they need. It's hurting both the patient and business. With that firmly in mind, I might ask a couple of questions like this:

Q2. Let's talk more about patient objections, and specifically, why people say 'no' to physical therapy even though they need it:

a. Tell me about a situation when a patient, even though they needed physical therapy, didn't want to commit. What was their reason and how did you handle it?

b. Other than cost, what other reasons for reluctant attendance have you heard from patients who need physical therapy?

c. How did you overcome those objections?

d. How, specifically, have you handled situations where you know that a patient needs physical therapy, yet they tell you it's too expensive?

e. Tell me about a time when a patient needed more treatment, but their insurance did not cover it; how did you get the patient to agree to pay out of pocket/in cash?

f. What would be your specific strategy be to win back a patient who dropped off from your program?

These types of questions are drastically overlooked, yet they are taking you to the heart of the candidate's ability to solve a huge problem in most clinics these days. I'd be pretty sure that not being able to find someone with great clinical skills doesn't keep you awake at night. Instead, it's not being able to find someone who can keep your patients on schedule that does!

WHY I DON'T SPEND TOO MUCH TIME ON QUESTIONS ABOUT CLINICAL SKILLS

You might be thinking, "but Paul, where are all of the questions about clinical skills?" Well, I personally don't ask too many of them.

I've never had to fire or let go of a therapist simply because their clinical skills were not up to scratch. I've always let physical therapists go because they were *unable to communicate* in a way that ensured a patient actually stuck around long enough to feel the benefit of their skills. At times, they were simply unwilling to execute this vital task; they thought it was beneath them to have to talk to a patient in fourth grade language.

However, just because someone has an expensive qualification or a doctorate level degree, it does not automatically mean that people can instantly understand what it means enough to want to pay to access the skills that come with it; no, you still have to communicate the value of what it means and it takes being able to communicate radically different than most are ever taught in PT School.

Sadly, not every physical therapist is willing to stomach that and it is to their own, the patients, and the professions, detriment.

I also know from experience working with business owners from all over the world – hundreds, heading towards thousands – that not one of them has ever had an issue with a physical therapist's lack of clinical skills. But, I know a large majority who have employed great clinicians with amazing skills, but can't talk to people. They simply cannot explain why their patients need to come for all of the nine sessions that were prescribed.

Conversely, I've met many business owners who tell me that the *least* clinically skilled person in their practice – often the newest – is frequently pulling in the best numbers (completed plans of care and patient visit average, etc.).

I'm not suggesting that clinical skills are irrelevant; I am suggesting that many clinic owners make the mistake of thinking that a better or more skilled clinician is what they want – and even when they get what they want, they still fire or let them go because they can't keep people on schedule!

All the clinical skills in the world won't solve the problem if the patient doesn't know why they need to show up more than they thought they would need to.

That's where the problems come in and this is yet another example of hiring to solve the wrong problem.

If it is that important to you to see some evidence of clinical skills before you hire, what you might consider doing is some kind of trial. Start by setting up five patients who you know. Ask a friend who needs help, or that family member who always wants to ask you about their health problems, and have the candidate treat them.

Get some feedback from each one those patients and use it to validate or confirm your thoughts; don't hire or discount them just because your favorite Aunt Sally liked the person. Take what those people say and add it to the profile of the candidate you are building.

RUN OVER THE HOMEWORK TASK

Once I've probed deeper with my focused questions, I let the candidate present their homework task to me. This is the point in the interview that I really look forward to. That's because the candidate is about to start teaching me something about how to better solve the problems in my business (I hope!).

Don't look at the interview process as just being about what you can learn about the candidate. You should also consider what you might learn from them. If you go into every situation looking to learn from it, then guess what, you usually do! This is true in all aspects of business and life – not just hiring.

What's more, the homework task often creates a situation for spontaneous dialogue. And that's important, because it allows you to find out even more about what they do or do not know.

As they talk to me, I have another opportunity to ask more questions on the subject that I wasn't planning to ask – so they're very unlikely to have prepared "canned" responses. As well as what they are telling me, I am also looking for visual clues. How comfortable are they? Is their body language relaxed? Are they breathing calmly, or is the color draining from the candidate's cheeks? Or, are they uptight and anxious, wanting to rush the presentation as fast as possible due to lack of knowledge?

Again, none of these things guarantee getting someone the position (or losing him or her the position), they are all just clues helping me to build a case to find the right candidate.

GIVE CANDIDATES THE OPPORTUNITY TO ASK QUESTIONS

I like to finish every interview by giving the candidate the opportunity to ask me some questions. I'm hoping they'll ask me about what makes my company so special, something about why my current staff enjoys working for me. Maybe they'll ask what the next step in the company's growth is, or how this role will evolve with it? If they do, I know I'm talking to someone who is looking for things I can provide. These are much better questions than the usual, "what time will I start?", and they say so much more about the candidate.

This is also my license to really sell the company, the role, and myself to them – <u>again</u>! I am going to go into overdrive and make the company and the role sound more appealing than I ever could have in a written ad. That's not just because I'm passionate about my companies, or because I believe in what I am saying, it's because I know that this is my last chance to increase the candidate's desire to work for me.

I cannot overstate how important it is that you sell **you**.

This affects how candidates see you, how they respect you, how motivated they are, and how likely they are to, not just accept your job offer, but be thrilled to do so. There's a difference. Having your staff buy into who they are working for is huge. Remember ultimately, they are coming to work for you, not your company.

You must display an energy, a passion, and a love for what you've created and what you do. It needs to be visible.

It needs to be felt, so don't hold back from displaying it. People are desperate to be in the presence of someone who has an energy that can be felt; it makes them feel much better about themselves! It makes it easier to get out of bed each day if they know they're going to be around someone with passion, energy, and enthusiasm for what they do. It is a rare thing these days. If you've got it, show it off and don't hold back.

I am 100% certain that doing this has allowed me to win the decision of some of my best staff – some of whom, at the time of interviewing with me, also had other offers on the table. I am also 100% certain that it's allowed me to recruit those same staff for a salary that was less than they were being offered elsewhere at the same time.

Despite what you might want to believe, money is not the only thing that factors in to whether or not people want to work for you. The person that they will be working for, and the environment that they'll be working in, is often worth taking a pay cut for.

THE IDEAL SITUATION - A SLEEPLESS NIGHT!

Ok, so I've interviewed the final three or four candidates, and the ideal situation is that I'm "torn" between at least two of them. I'm hoping to be able to have a *sleepless night* after the final day of interviews.

I want to be in a situation where I'm literally dreading having to tell one of the candidates that they didn't get the job.

In theory, the <u>worst-case</u> scenario is that there is a clear-cut winner. That is because it could mean that the other three performed really badly, and I don't want to be hiring someone just because the other three didn't perform (remember, this was one of the mistakes from chapter 2).

I never want to be in a position where I am hiring someone just because the others were underwhelming. And funnily enough, just a month or so before I started writing this book, that type of thing happened to me.

True story: I was looking for a new staff member for my marketing company, *Paul Gough Media*. This is the business that provides marketing and business training to physical therapy business owners all across the world; we've grown so fast in the last couple of years that I'm nearly always adding new people to the team. This was my fifth addition to the team in six months, and the role was for someone to provide an additional level of customer service and support to the members of our **Cash Club** Program (details here: www.ptprofitacadey.com/cash-club).

Cash Club is a program that helps new and fledgling business owners start learning more from me. It helps them learn more about what it takes to market and run a successful physical therapy clinic. And, because we offer one-on-one support to members, the role required the candidate to have prior experience in working with people, handling customer accounts, talking at length to customers, building relationships, and having an understanding of just what it is like to run a small business.

In this case, I did everything that I have so far described in this book; I ran the ads, I attracted the candidates, and I carried out the interviews as documented herein. It was going so well right up until the point when I had two of my final three drop out of the race.

Both of the candidates who dropped out were from the same company. It seems that both used my role, and my interest in them, as a pawn to secure themselves a better situation in their current role. So, in this particular situation, I now only had one candidate to interview. Of course, I did the interview and I was impressed.

But, and it's a huge *but*, I had no one to compare the girl who was interviewed to. So, how did I know how good she really was? I had no frame of reference. When you purchase a house, you only know that the one you got is the perfect one for you because you compared it to five others.

It's the same with business and financials – how do you know you've had a good or a bad year, really? Because that year is compared to the three previous years, and in this way you're able to come to a conclusion based on data and trends. It has to be the same with hiring.

Despite having a situation in which I desperately needed to fill the role (because we had more new members of Cash Club coming in daily), I decided to start the process all over again.

I politely explained to the candidate what the situation was – and what my reasoning was; that I thought she was great, but I had no one to compare her to. I realize that this would sound strange to most people, and anyone the girl told would have said I was a just messing with her – but, I wasn't. I was following a process. And the reason I follow the process is because every single time I've violated the rules I've set in business, I always get stung.

I re-started the ads, we attracted more candidates, and that resulted in three more people making their way to the focused interview. Four weeks later I had the right person. It <u>wasn't</u> the girl from the first round of interviews. Turns out that first girl was good – and would have done the job ok – but the person I got was a significantly better skilled and a more suitable candidate, and I was happy I waited to find her.

Moral of the story? Follow the process no matter what the circumstances.

PICK ONE — KEEP IT RIGHT WITH THE OTHER

Once you've picked your no.1 candidate, it's important to consider the ones you're going to say no to. I recommend that you think long and hard about how to tell the person you didn't pick, <u>why</u> you didn't pick them.

You need to find that one stand out feature or benefit that the person you chose had, but which the candidate you didn't pick, lacked.

What's more, explain your decision in a way that helps them truly understand the reasoning behind it. It wasn't that the other candidate was more qualified or more experienced, it was that they had something that you were specifically looking for, and that was what got them the role.

For example, I remember explaining, to one particular candidate, that the only reason I'd given the other person a job was because he knew a particular software that I use (Infusionsoft) better than anyone I'd ever interviewed. With everything else equal, this got him the role. But, I also explained that I would love to give the un-hired candidate a job as soon as the next position comes up in the office.

This is vital to do, because even though you're confident and happy with the person you picked, there's a still a chance it might not go according to plan. The reason you wanted to have a sleepless night over two people is because it means you have a plan B to go to if A doesn't work out.

How you communicate, and how well you protect the relationship with plan B, will determine whether or not they're still interested in coming to work for you later on (if A doesn't work out).

Another reason that you want two equally skilled candidates at the end is so that you are in control of the process. I once hired someone using this exact process, who, when I offered the candidate a job, asked me for a higher salary than I was originally offering.

I was un-phased when I categorically said I would not be able to do it. I wasn't worried about losing the candidate, because I had a plan B.

Here's the thing: it wasn't that the person I was offering the role to wasn't worth what she was asking – she was and is – it's just that I had a process and I needed to stick to it. Because I had a plan B, it meant I wasn't worried in the slightest if the person said no to me; plan B was waiting in the wings.

Everything that I do in business – and subsequently teach you – is about stacking the odds of success in **your** favor so that you never have to feel like you're making decisions out of sheer desperation.

Which, sadly, is the norm for most business owners. Yet, it really doesn't have to be that way. Follow the right frameworks, allocate the necessary time, and think carefully over the consequences of your decisions before you rush into them. Do that and you'll find yourself making a lot more good decisions, rather than bad ones. It's not sexy – but it sure is effective.

PART 4: MEET THE TEAM

So, you've made your decision. You've picked your candidate, and the next thing that you could do is have your team confirm everything that you've so far seen. Can they validate the decision that you've already made?

Truth be told, I don't always do this, but I have done it, and I've seen it done by many people, so I wanted to share it with you.

Think of it as an extra layer of protection against you making the wrong decision, or, confirming that you've made the right decision.

The scenario is this: you've chosen the person who you believe to be your current first choice. Do not tell the candidate this, and likewise, don't tell your staff. Just tell them that you're very interested in this candidate and you want to know what they think of the person in terms of personality and values.

You then tell the candidate that are they very close to getting the role and that you want them to meet the rest of the team. Tell the candidate that this is to make sure they would be happy working with your team should you offer them the job.

Now, what you do next is this: don't tell anyone on your team anything about what you believe to be the strengths and weaknesses of the candidate. Do not allow bias to creep into the situation. Let your staff take this person out for lunch and spend a couple of hours with the candidate; let them get to know the candidate so that they can get their own insight into who this person is. They're not looking for proof of skills – they're just getting a feel for if this person would be someone who could/would fit nicely into the team, culturally.

Once they've spent time with the candidate, get together with your team and find out what they think.

Is what they are telling you what you saw in the interview? Does it confirm your profile? Are there any alarm bells ringing with anyone? Did the candidate let slip anything that you didn't find out?

This strategy is a great way of separating two superstars if you really can't choose between them. And, it's an equally great way of confirming that you've made the right decision. What it also does is further empower your team; it proves to the candidate that you are the type of person who values and respects the opinion of your staff. That is only going to do you good when it comes to them accepting your offer.

PART 5: CHECK REFERENCES

There's a lot of debate over whether or not to check references. After all, who is going to put down a reference that would say something bad about them?

And what's more, you have to factor in that legally, and in most places, referees are not allowed to say anything bad about a candidate if it might cost them a job.

It is madness, but that is the way this crazy world is headed. This is a world in which everyone except the business owner has rights; a world where a previous boss cannot give their thoughts on an employee – who, despite being paid every month, was late regularly, regularly missed deadlines, turned up hung-over, disrupted company culture, or wasn't able to carry out simple tasks because they were too busy messing around on social media during work hours. It's sad, but that's the way it is. And what is worse, the governments actually think that they're doing the employees a favor.

At best, get clever with your questions to references and ask things of previous employers, like: "So that I can support this person best, in what areas could I help this person improve or develop?", or, "what are the areas that you think I should focus on to help them become even better at what they can do?"

Look at the questions again; inadvertently, you're asking the referee to tell you where the candidate's weaknesses are. It's like I said earlier, the quality of your questions determines the quality of your answers.

Final point: look for clues in their work history; if there are obvious gaps in recent jobs – and they have not been travelling around the world for a few years – then it's because the candidate doesn't want you to know where they've worked. The question is, why don't they want you to know? Make it your job to find that out.

PART 6: MAKE THE OFFER AND NEGOTIATE

The last thing to do is make the offer. And what is more, be prepared to negotiate. I'm not going to get into the particulars of what you offer (pay, 401K, health insurance, etc.), as every situation is different.

However, at the higher level what you need to do is offer whatever you need to get the outcome you want; however, you should only pay within the limits of what you can realistically afford to pay so that you don't risk the business or put it in danger.

Don't be afraid to start your offer low; as I've said already, people are *not* solely motivated by a higher salary. Only a boss who is absent of leadership skills, people skills or a culture that is a pleasure to work in, will tell you otherwise. Many things determine why someone will accept or decline a job. Not just pay.

If the person you want has previously earned a higher salary elsewhere, so what? It doesn't mean that they were happy; the cost of the commute, or two hours lost sitting in rush hour traffic every day, is probably not worth the additional $10k that they are currently being paid.

I've had many people take a "pay cut" in their gross salary to come and work for me. I say gross because although on paper, it might say $35k in their current salary, by the time they pay $5k in gas and $2k in parking…then they factor in needing to leave the house an hour earlier and arriving back home an hour later (meaning they lose ten hours a week with their kids), taking a $28k role with me that is five minutes from their house is all of a sudden, very attractive.

And the smart employees know it; when they calculate the cost of sitting in their car for two hours every day, they soon realize the hourly rate that is on offer from you is significantly more than they are currently making. With all of these things considered, it's no wonder they're happy to take a "cut."

The other lesson I wanted to pass on to you is this: don't be frightened to negotiate. It doesn't mean that you have a bad candidate just because they want more. It might actually mean you have someone with other options; it might mean you have someone confident about themselves and who is looking for the absolute best that they can get. Why wouldn't they? If you're offering them lower than they want, you're doing exactly the same; you're simply trying to get the best for yourself. And so you should.

Please bare this in mind – it doesn't make them a bad candidate if they want to negotiate, it just means they want to make sure they get the best for themselves. Conversely, it doesn't make you a bad boss if you want to pay less; it just means that you want to get the best for yourself. As long as you can both find common ground in the end, and both parties are happy, then you've made a fair deal that is more likely to see both parties happy in the long run and the employee last.

Ideally, you've got options like I had in the situation that I described earlier; with a plan B in place I was in a win-win situation so I didn't feel the need to negotiate. However, if you're not in that situation, don't be afraid to do it. I wouldn't be.

Ok, so you've picked your stand-out candidate, the reference checks are done, and the negotiation has ended well for both of you. The hiring process doesn't stop there, though.

Next up you've got to give the newly hired person the best possible shot at being successful in the role. That involves an onboarding process that prepares your new hire for how you want them to perform in the role.

We'll cover that in the next chapter. Turn the page and let's get going...

11

YOUR FOOLPROOF 7, 30 AND 90 DAY ONBOARDING PROCESS

You've picked your player, now you have to on-board them. That involves a mix of training and coaching. What is the difference? *Training* is telling someone exactly what to do. You're often teaching them something from scratch. *Coaching* is optimizing what they've learned. As a business owner, I try to spend more time coaching than training. I leave my senior staff to the training and then I get involved later when it is time to optimize what the new member has learned. Of course, if it's your first hire you're going to have to do both.

Despite everything that we've just covered, I firmly believe that what happens next is the one single thing that will determine how successful this person is going to be.

Tip: what you do from now on is perhaps more important than what they do. If you abdicate the tasks required of this person, without first making sure they are able to perform, then you'll be setting this person up for failure.

With that in mind, I've created a 90-day "fool proof" onboarding system that I want to share with you. It is broken up into four distinct parts which provide guidelines for the training and coaching you'll need to do or oversee.

We'll look at the first 7, 30, and 90 days – and then, how you'll continue to optimize thereafter. What happens in the first 7 days is usually more important than what happens in the first 30, and what happens in the first 30 is more important than what happens in the first 90 days.

As you think about on-boarding your new employee, it's important to tie all of their training and coaching back to my favorite document – the *Success Description*. Think about it, everything that you were hiring for is written down on that document. Therefore, everything that you need the person to do (now that you have hired them) is contained within that document, and it is going to act as your point of reference for how you'll work with your new employee moving forward.

Said differently, the reason that most people struggle to know what to do when it comes to onboarding their new hire is because they didn't have a *Success Description*, clearly outlining what they need to be trained for!

WHAT HAPPENS IN THE FIRST 7 DAYS

So, what does happen in the first 7 days? The answer is, whatever your *Success Description* has deemed to be the most important tasks.

In the first 7 days, I like to make sure that the candidate understands the most important one or two aspects of their role. Ideally, by the end of week one they've been trained and *are* now doing it.

I've made so many mistakes in hiring, and one of them is to put off the bigger, more important tasks, thinking that it's better to let the candidate ease their way into the role. In my opinion, this is a mistake. That is because whatever you start training on, or whatever you introduce to them first, is what they believe to be their most important role. After that, when you try to introduce new things to them, they'll always put those off tin order to ensure that the first things you showed them get done promptly.

I see this happening all the time, especially when the business owner starts to learn new ways of doing things. At first it was all about sending off bills to insurance companies or paper work being done correctly. Then later, when the owner tries to get them to do things like patient callbacks or using a new script, the employee seems reluctant to do it. They always default to those first things, and these are often the transactional things that don't really make that much of a difference to your outcomes.

The other reason I want to get straight into important tasks first is because I do not want to make it easy initially.

I don't want to lure them into a false sense of complacency, as though my place is a cushy place to work.

When a new member of staff arrives it's easy for everyone to want to concentrate on being "liked". It's a natural human reaction to want to be liked by someone at work, so it leads to people changing or temporarily modifying the way they behave. Most importantly, it leads to a change in the way they communicate. Tony Robbins talks about "softeners", a language pattern that people adopt when they want to make a good first impression.

This "softening" happens in both interviews and when people first arrive at work. We tend to soften what we say so that we don't come across as abrupt, stern, or arrogant. And, as a result, believe someone will like us more for doing so. For example, "are you ok to stay back late to finish this training?" is what you might say on day 1.

But, four months in you're likely to say, "we ARE staying back late tonight to finish this training."

We do it with patients, too. Instead of telling them how many sessions they need, and exactly what it's going to cost, clinicians will often say something softer like, "let's have a few sessions and see how it goes". There's nothing uncomfortable about that type of conversation, but it really isn't helping anyone get what they want. It feels nice at the time, but long term it's bad for both patient and clinic – it's a conversation lacking certainty.

There's a fine line to draw when you speak to a new employee in the early phase of their employment. You do not want to come across as a militant, but at the same time you don't want to come across as though you're someone you're not; you can't keep the soft approach up forever.

How will they react when you go back to being a little more stern or abrupt?

So, for me, the first 7 days are really about getting them competent in the most important couple of tasks in the role. Here are a few specific examples:

THE FIRST 7 DAYS FOR A FRONT DESK PERSON

Let's look back at the *Success Description* that I created for the front desk person. One of the things that I want this person to be able to do is ensure names appear on the schedule. If people are calling and they're suitable for what we do, I want to see them scheduled.

Now, for that to happen, one of the tasks that they'll have to be able to do successfully is handle price objections. That was listed in my *Success Description* as, "successfully handle price objections". For them to be able to do this, I will need to walk the employee through precisely how I want each objection handled.

Ideally, I want them to do it in the exact same way that *I've* successfully been handling it in the last few months, or years, before they were hired.

Just because this person is good on the phone, is confident, or even that they've been able to handle price objections in their previous role, it does not mean they can handle the *"do you take my insurance?"* question in the same way that I've done, a way that is proven to be the most successful.

"TALK, SHOW, DO" - THE SIMPLE 3-STEP PROCESS FOR TRAINING

I'm going to prioritize the, *"do you take my insurance"* question, because we hear it all the time. If my new hire gets asked it five times in week one, and they can't deal with it, that could cost me close to $10,000. That is significantly more than I would be paying them, and so the real cost of *not* training employees is *not* what you pay them, it's what you lose when you pay them while expecting them to perform just because you are paying them.

I use a simple 3-step process that you could follow; I call it "talk, show, do". Here's how it works:

1. TALK THEM THROUGH IT

On the very first day, talk them through how you want them to handle the major 4 or 5 objections that will come up. Ideally, you'll have some training videos pre-made for them to watch, and if you haven't, start the process of recording all of the training sessions with this person.

It makes sense on so many levels. Not just because it allows the person to go back over it and listen to the session (to hear things that they missed, or to gain a deeper understanding of the things they did hear), but also because, and here's the best part, it makes future recruiting so much easier.

When you start creating a library of training videos, it allows your staff to do most of their own training. You are not relinquishing control, in fact, you are leveraging your time. If I have taught it in a way that I am happy with – and it's recorded – then what is wrong with me giving that video to every new member of my staff on morning one of their employment? Until your understanding of the issue changes, or you find a better way, the current version is good enough to hand over.

At this point I am not expecting the new employee to 100% understand what I want them to do. But, after watching a training video (while you are busy doing something else), it allows you to go back to the person and, quite literally, fill in the blanks. The best teachers do not really "teach", they fill in the knowledge gaps. They start by asking, "what do you already know about this subject?", and they then proceed to go deeper or fill in holes.

It is no different with employees. To avoid wasting time, you want to find out what they currently don't know, then you want to work with them and take them to a point where they do know (what they need to know). Recordings and videos are a great way for you to do this.

2. SHOW THEM HOW TO DO IT

So, on the first day (Monday) I've **talked** through what I want the new employee to do. I may have gone over a script or role-played it with them (which I thoroughly encourage you to do – regularly). So the next thing I am going to do (perhaps the next day; Tuesday) is **show** them how to do it.

I might start the training session with a re-cap of what the employee picked up from the training the day before. I'll answer any questions or fill in the blanks before I give a demonstration on how to do it.

At this point, I am showing them how *I* would handle the objection.

In this instance, I'll have them listen into a call that I handle (use a speaker phone) and have them critique me when I finish. The best way to learn is to teach, so if you reverse the process at this point – have them explain to you why the call was good (or bad!) – you will really help them to synthesize their knowledge. This will make it so much easier for the employee to execute when it is their turn.

3. THEY DO IT FOR THEMSELVES

The next day (it is now day 3 – perhaps Wednesday), you're going to ask them to do it themselves. The key point here that you must understand (and that the employee must also understand), is that they are not being judged on the outcome of the call, only the fact that the call took place.

Change the metric of success from a patient scheduling, to them just actually doing it (making the call).

This gives them what I call a "little win" – a feeling of accomplishment that is important in the first few days of being hired. Even if the call doesn't end well, that's ok. The fact that the call took place is what matters at this stage. Of course, if they keep making the call and the patients don't schedule, then that is a different thing altogether.

But, that'll come up in your review of the measurable outcomes later in the process.

THE FIRST 7 DAYS FOR A PHYSICAL THERAPIST

Next, let's look at an example of the first 7 days for a physical therapist.

Going back to the *Success Description* we created in Chapter 7, one of the tasks that I prioritized for my new physical therapist is ensuring that a new patient converts from a first session to a plan of care; following that first session, they come back and have more.

Why is this important? Well, if the therapist can't get this right, (and quickly), you're going to be losing a lot of money. What's more, almost everything else is irrelevant; if the patient doesn't come back after the first session then there's no NPS score, there's not going to be any completed plan of care ratio to look at, and there won't be any notes completed on time. There's always one thing that supersedes everything else, and in the case of the physical therapist, this is it. That's why I focus on it in the first week.

I'm going to follow the **"talk, show, do"** process that I described above.

On the Monday, I might talk them about how I do it; I'll give the physical therapist tips for communicating with a patient in a way that makes them want to say yes to us. And, I'll also explain how I package up treatment sessions.

I insist on my therapists offering packages to my patients. I do not ever want the patient to walk out unsure of how many sessions, in total, they're going to need to get better. Offering packages is vital to both the running of my business and the patients health. Having done it many times over, I'll explain the common questions I get from people in the first session, and I'll even discuss objections to booking packages. If I have videos, then I am having them watch these videos as well, and if I don't, I'm starting to record them at the same time.

The next day, I'll let the physical therapist watch me (or someone else in the team) do an initial evaluation. I'll have them watch me and afterwards, critique my performance. At the end of the session, I'll have them describe what they saw; I want to know if what I told the therapist in the meeting (the day before) matched up to what I actually did. Did the therapist see what I told them?

Tip: you should allocate 30 minutes directly after that session to review it with them. Use this time to reconfirm the major principles of what you expect in tomorrow's session, which is when they will be doing it.

On day 3, it's now the physical therapist's turn to do it. And much like the front of house person, the only metric of success is that they actually do it. At this point you're not judging the new employee, you're just observing and helping. That's why you should sit in on the session with them no matter how uncomfortable they may feel about it.

THE CULTURAL INDOCTRINATION

As well as picking one or two major tasks from the *Success Description*, in the first week I also like the employee to experience what I term a "cultural indoctrination". This is when the new hire gets to know everyone else in my team, personally and professionally. I want my new hire to find out what everyone else in my team does and what their outcomes are.

Each day on the first week I will allocate time for this new employee to talk to another member of staff. It could be one hour, maybe two. The goal is finding out what the new person thinks is the other persons role in the business. I then ask the new employee to relay it back to me; do they understand how what others do, will impact what they will be doing for me?

Doing this also allows for the people in your business to get to know each other on a personal level. This is in addition to understanding one of the most important aspects of the business – how they're all working together to serve your patients.

I've found that, if employees can truly understand what the purposes of each other's roles are, then the compound effect of their roles is felt much more strongly by the patient.

When they each understand what they're all doing, it is much easier to make a collective impact; this impact is felt more strongly by the patient, and in a way that no single person could ever make on his or her own.

By doing this you're already starting to make the business the sum of all its parts, and this is the only way to rid yourself of ever feeling like you need to depend upon one "rock star".

How to do it? Simply have your new employee spend an hour with each different employee. Let them ask questions about patients, the major objectives of the company, a little history, and that employee's view of working for the company. I even go so far as to ask them to find out more about <u>me</u>.

That's right, I want the current employees telling the new employees what I am really like; not who I think I am, or who I've been through the recruitment process, but who I am on a consistent day-to-day basis. This is massively important, as it is sending more signals that you've got nothing to hide and that the new employee has nothing to fear by working for you. I'm still selling the role to them long after they accepted.

Another thing I do – and this is perfect if you are recruiting your first staff person – is have a new employee get on the phone to patients.

Have them talk to your patients about what they love about your clinic and have them ask what the patients love about coming to see you. The new employee should be looking for clues on how to perform to keep your best patients happy.

The call is simply a "fact find", and the only real objective is to connect and engage with your best patients. This is strengthening the relationship the business has with them.

<u>First of all</u>, it puts the employee at ease. It is something they can do very easily without any pressure or worry of getting it wrong. What's more, if your new hire asks the right questions, it's actually going to reveal a lot about you as an employer that you want your patient to hear.

Think about it, if the employee picks up the phone in the first week, with the aim of introducing themselves to 50 of your best patients (10 per day), then there is going to be many good things said about you by the patients. This will further reinforce the employee's decision to want to work for you.

Remember, it's not just the employee on trial at this point – you are too.

If they hear 50 people saying amazing things about you, then they get the feel-good factor that comes with working for a place/someone who is well liked. They'll (hopefully) feel an overwhelming amount of love for you coming from your patients, and it'll immediately elevate the respect that the new hire has for you.

I always say there's a big difference between working for someone and *wanting* to work for someone; the people who you can trust are those who *want* to work for you, and doing this lets the person believe, and feel for themselves, that you're a great person to want to work for.

<u>Why else</u> do I like having new staff pick up the phone to patients? It's because you'll also land a few patients in the process.

Depending on the size of your patient database, there could literally be dozens, or hundreds, of your past patients who should come back and see you.

Right now, you've got past patients who keep forgetting to book. They have nagging back or neck pain that's been there for weeks. When they get this call from your new staff person they will actually do it (book in). If you get 5 people to come back and see you, and your average patient spends $1,000 with you, you've just covered the employee's first few months' salary. Not to mention, you've created a lot of good will in your clinic.

It's for all those reasons that I love to get my staff on the phone to patients quickly, and you could do this with both a front desk person and a physical therapist. It is a simple, "hello, I am new around here – tell me what you love about the clinic so that I can continue to meet the standards that have been set before me". This is not that difficult for anyone to do, and yet the rewards are huge.

THE ESSENTIALS – HR, BILLING SOFTWARE, HEALTH AND SAFETY

Last, but not least, within the first seven days you're obviously going to do all of the logistical and legal necessaries. You'll explain the HR policy, show the new hire the health and safety file, where the fire door is, how the vacation request process works, when they paid, how to lock up and close, passwords, billing software, and so on and so on.

Most people are already doing something like this and, of course, they're important. But, this is not nearly as important as picking one major task and starting the process of mastering it, as well as setting up a solid cultural indoctrination involving getting to know staff and patients.

FIRST 30 DAYS FOR A FRONT DESK PERSON

This phase is about assessing your new employee's current level of competence in the major tasks you identified. That's because your chance to measure how well they are doing comes at the end of the first 30 days.

After 30 days, you want them to have been doing most of the major tasks. And that's because you can then have your first objective look at their performance and your coaching.

Remember, this is a two-way thing; for athletes to prosper, they need a great coach. It is the same in business. For your people to become star people, how much you develop and coach them will determine the heights they can reach.

Now at this point, you're not making any snap judgments about the person, you're just measuring where they currently are. You're going to look closely at the measurable outcomes that you set for them (when you hired them), and measure those against where they are currently performing.

If you're asking for an 80% conversion ratio from phone call to patient, and the person is at 20%, then you would be right to be concerned.

However, if the data is telling you that the current level of performance is at 70%, then that's ok. That, to me, would be an acceptable level of performance. It would be enough evidence to suggest that I can work with this person to get them closer to the 80% standard that I expect.

To sum up, this phase is about continuing to work with and coach your employee. It could be as little as 30 minutes per day, or as much as four hours per day, on the specific tasks we talked about in the *Success Description*. The tasks that when you hit the standard is going to make a big difference to the profitability of your business.

FIRST 90 DAYS FOR A FRONT DESK PERSON

You're now getting to the point where you're starting to see (objectively) just how good this person is. Throughout the last 90 days you should have been working and improving on all of the tasks identified in the tasks section of the *Success Description*. What's more, you should have gone through two lots of performance measuring (30 and 60 days) and should now be close to getting an accurate idea of how capable they are.

Ideally, at this point we want to have seen their standards improve month over month:

FIG.12

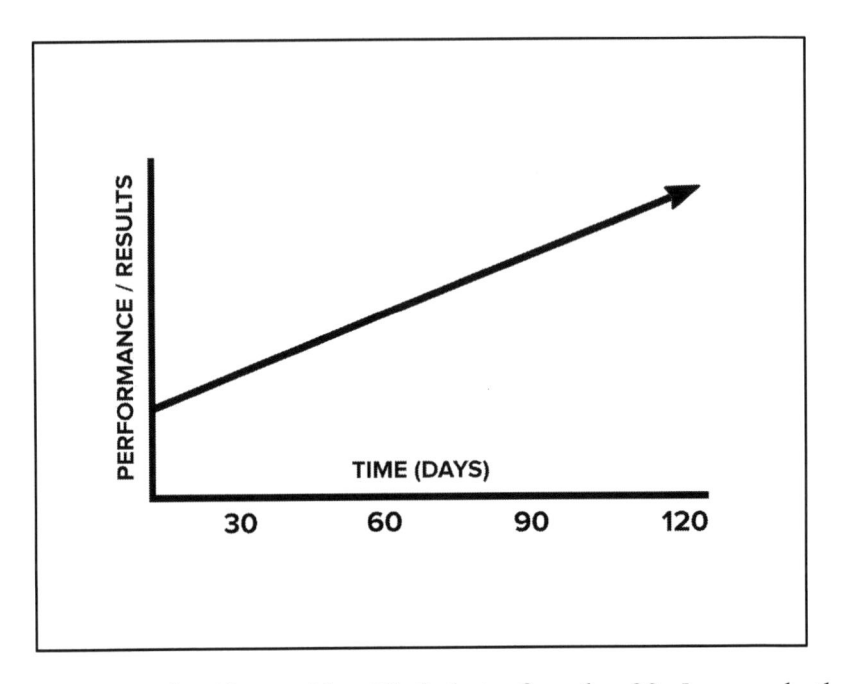

[Graph showing an upward trending line with PERFORMANCE / RESULTS on the y-axis and TIME (DAYS) on the x-axis, with markers at 30, 60, 90, and 120 days]

For example, if you identified that after the **30 day** mark their standards were at **60%** conversion to paying patient, and that at **60 days** it was at **70%**, then what you're hoping for at 90 days is for it to be at **80%** – this is the agreed standard of performance required to achieve the outcome you hired for.

FIRST 90 DAYS FOR A PHYSICAL THERAPIST

For your physical therapist, you're following the same rules: continue to train, monitor, and optimize all of the key tasks you outlined in the *Success Description*. By now you should have gone through multiple rounds of training on how to do the major tasks, such as, for example, converting from Discovery visits to a full plan of care, or ensuring a Net Promoter Score of above 8.

Basically, they should now be well on their way to hitting the required standards.

TIME TO MAKE A DECISION

This is a crucial point in the hiring process; it's at this point that you're going to be making a big decision about the employee's future. Should they stay or should they go?

Everything we've done so far is about putting you in a situation where you are able to make an objective judgment about the performance of the person you've hired. A lot of people can interview well, but it is at this time that the "proof is in the pudding", as I like to say.

Now that you've seen them in action, you can ask yourself, "is this person who you need?". "Can this person solve your problem?" By now, you should have the data to back it up and find you answer.

Earlier in the book, I wrote about the importance of having all of your employees hired with a 90-day probation in their contract. This allows both parties to exit the relationship if it is not working out. If you do everything that I've told you to do so far in this book, it is impossible to be saddled with an employee that isn't right for you.

If you have measured their performance, and you have a 90-day exit clause in place, it stops you from getting into a long-term commitment with someone who is not capable. Think of this point as a junction in the road; currently the lights are red, forcing you to think about what direction you're going to go in next. Doing this means you'll need to lift your head from out of the day-to-day running of the business and reflect on how good this person actually is. You should be taking some time to consider all of the facts, and you should be asking yourself if the employee has lived up to the promise shown in the interview – or not.

What happens next is going to be based on what the data is telling you. If you haven't been measuring their performance, and you do not have an objective measure to refer to, then you're going off of your gut. And what is the biggest hiring mistake? That's right, going off your gut (refer back to chapter 2). If all you rely on at this stage is your emotions, then the likelihood of getting it right is slim.

If they're not performing as well as you hoped, take the time to consider why. Were you overly optimistic with your standards? Was this the first hire you've made, and did you set the outcomes too high? That is possible. In that case, you need to consider, if the employee keeps performing at the current level, can you make the profit you want?

It is possible that the current level of performance is less than you had hoped for, but that the employee is still able to bring in the level of profit you want.

What we've done with the framework and focus on outcomes is put you in a position to make a better decision.

If you make better decisions, you'll have a better business.

If the employee's performance is down, is it because you didn't allocate the appropriate training? Is it your fault? You need to ask yourself if you provided the right level of support and training, and if not, do you need to extend their probation and this time do it right? From this far off, I obviously can't know the answers. But, I do know that the framework I've given you will guide you to them.

All of these things must be considered before you make the decision. Use the data in conjunction with your subjective view to determine what happens next.

It can never be your subjective view on its own. The subjective view is quick and easy. It is also what gets you into a lot of trouble… and is also why so many businesses are shackled with dead-beat employees who are holding them back.

STUNNINGLY SIMPLE

As you can see, this is an incredibly simple, and radically logical, process for hiring and on-boarding successfully. And *that* is going to be the problem for most who are reading this, as there's a big difference between common sense and common practice. The latter requires the work is done and that the framework is followed.

You've just been given a step-by-step system for finding people you can trust. Will you execute all that you've learned, or will you take short cuts when the busy-ness of running a business gets in the way?

Here's a thought: why do so many business owners get dragged into the "busy-ness" of their business, anyway? It's because of poorly performing or inept staff. How did they get there in the first place? Because of bad hiring decisions.

Think about it – when was the last time you put out a fire you started? When was the last time you were called to fix something that you didn't do properly? When was the last time you didn't show up for work?

The reason that business owners will try to skip parts of this process is the exact reason they need to do the *entire* process.

If you do (complete the process), you'll see stunning results. The absolute worst that can happen is, at the 90 days mark, you'll be showing someone where the exit door is because they couldn't perform. Better that though than carrying a dead weight. Carry too many dead weights and, after a while, you'll sink.

Ideally, we don't want to show someone the door, but even if it does need to happen, this system will have been a success. That is because the absolute worst thing that can happen is that a bad employee actually *hangs around*. It will cost you a lot more to keep one than to let one go – no matter how much time you've invested in the process.

ON-GOING WEEKLY TRAINING AND COACHING

Assuming that the new hire makes it to day 91, the final piece in the onboarding process is the regular training and coaching.

Just because they've performed well up until now doesn't mean it will stay that way. There's no star performer anywhere who doesn't need to be continuously trained and coached. Your employees are no different.

The level of disrespect for regular training that most business owners show amazes me. If you're not learning, you've plateaued. And if I'm the clinic owner across the street and my team and I *are* training and learning, then it's not going to be long before I overtake you.

The false belief is that the older you get, the wiser you get. That is one of the most ridiculous statements I've ever heard; only ever said by older people who didn't want to take the time to learn and grow. Here's the truth: if you're not learning, you're growing old, stupidly. If you're not getting coached, then you're not getting better.

There's a great saying that goes like this: "the chains of bad habits are often too soft to ever notice, yet too strong to ever break".

What this means is that bad habits will begin to creep into your employee's performance from the very first day you take your eye off of the ball. That means you can never do it.

One of the stupidest things that comes with adulthood is to think that because you're an adult, you're somehow exempt from the rules of how the brain wants to work - to do as little as it possibly can.

Your brain is the laziest organ in your body. It is designed to aid your survival and not much else. It is not designed to make you happy, or fulfilled, or anything else that people want without doing the work to get. It has the potential do those things, but only if you work at it – constantly.

If you don't, it will find ways to short cut things that you once did very well. It's when you take short cuts that you end up going the long way around.

I've seen this happen to members of my own staff. They start by following my script, and then one day they change it ever so slightly. They take out one word or change one question. Then, the next day they take out another word or ask a question I didn't ask them to.

Within a month they're having a completely different conversation than the one I taught them to have when they first arrived.

How did I know this was happening? Because the 90% conversion ratio to paying patient suddenly <u>dropped</u> to 60%. The objective measure is not the problem – that is the effect. The cause of the drop in new patient conversions was a <u>failure to follow the script</u>. That is the problem.

Every single one of us needs work, business owners included. Want to know why most businesses struggle? It's because of the owner; that they lack the **skills** to run a business. Why do they lack the skills? Because they don't get coached or trained on the skills they need. It is cause and effect.

I believe so strongly in the power of coaching that in my office we close for three hours every week. If you try to call my clinic on a Wednesday between 9am-12pm, there are twenty people in the building, but no one will answer the phone. That is because that time is dedicated solely to staff development and optimizing the performance of my assets.

If you tried to call my clinic to book an appointment, you'd likely get the voicemail. The accounts people might pick it up, but you wouldn't get through to my front desk people. The doors are locked, the blinds are pulled down, and all our attention is focused on how well we are currently working both individually and as a unit. Every week we're looking for gaps in performance, celebrating wins, role-playing phone calls and walk in situations, and always asking, "where can we get better?"

The physical therapists are involved too; they're working on a specific injury (relevant to our perfect patient population), talking through case studies, auditing each other's notes, and one of them is charged with doing a research-based presentation each week. The session will finish with some hands-on skill training (relevant to the topic that was presented), and thereafter everyone leaves a little smarter than when they arrived.

They also leave feeling energized and more optimistic, and a great team bond is being cemented.

This is also how you create a great culture. It doesn't just happen because you hire people with great personalities. It doesn't even happen when you pay them more money. Winning the lottery doesn't fix an unhappy marriage, and money doesn't fix cultural issues, either. Great cultures are formed when you hire people who want to do the things that create great cultures. And what are these things? Well, one of which, if not the most important, is valuing – and being constantly open to – learning and growing.

Now, if you think I am a little "mad" or "weird" for closing my clinic for three hours each week, then I think you're mad for *not* closing yours. I cannot understand how any business owner thinks it is acceptable not to be constantly training and developing their greatest asset – **their staff.**

Could you imagine the LA Lakers or the New York Yankees spending all their time playing the games and never sitting down to ask how they could improve? If the team that you follow did that, it wouldn't be long before you see their performance drop. Pretty soon you'd stop going to the game, as you wouldn't tolerate such inept performances in exchange for your hard earned money. Why is it ok at your office?

We might be closed for three hours. And you might be calculating that "cost" to you. But, I'd much rather lose 3 potential patients and, instead, focus more on being better for the other 50 who will call later that week. If you are that desperate for patients that you can't close for training, then it's a good sign that you're doing something wrong. Why not close for training to put it right?

You can call me stupid, but I know how impactful this has been for me. And what's more, my staff know it too.

They absolutely love the fact that I'm so committed to learning… and that's because I hired people who value the same thing. They also love that I'm prepared to put my money where my mouth is when it comes to the standards I expect. It's not just something that I say we'll do and then never follow through on.

I'm not always in the training, but my staff know full well that I am committed to learning and coaching; there is not a week that goes by where I'm not flying to a conference, on the phone to a business coach, or coming in and sharing something that I've learned from the latest book I've just finished reading. My point? If you want them to be enthusiastic about learning, you need to be enthusiastic about learning.

Everything that is good or bad about this wonderful business of yours will always come back to you and your standards. If you have not created a weekly training opportunity for your team, I urge you to consider it. The short-term loss is trivial in comparison to the long-term gain that you'll make.

On my 6-week online training program, *PT Business Growth School* (module 4), I go deeper into the exact regime for how we do this. An invitation to join the program is here: **www.paulsbgs.com**

DOES YOUR CALENDAR SUPPORT THE PLAN?

Before I finish this section, I couldn't end it without pointing this out: all of the above is fine in theory, but if your calendar does not reflect the time commitment required for doing this, then it is a complete waste of time.

If you're looking at this and thinking all of this is great, then that's because it is. But, so far it is all theory. The moment it moves from theory to *reality* is when it moves from a thought or idea held in your head, to an actionable item in your calendar.

One of the things I regularly ask the clinic owners in my *Mastermind Coaching* programs is this: "does your calendar reflect your priorities?"

What this means is that, if you're telling me that you want something to happen, but it doesn't appear in your calendar with an appropriate amount of time allocated, then it is not your priority. You have a wish list of things you hope will happen, but never will.

If you want this process to become a reality, it must be prioritized on your calendar. As you build out this on-boarding process for your employees, remember to consider the investment in time it will take to do it right.

If it's you doing it, block out time appropriately in order to provide the training and support we've discussed in this chapter. And if someone else is doing it, be sure to block off time for them too, and with the instruction that it is non-negotiable. Nothing will get in the way of it getting done no matter how big the fire appears to be in your clinic that day. If you do not do this, it'll never get done.

So, there you have it. There's your process for the initial on-boarding in the first 7, 30, and 90 days, as well as the non-stop optimizing of your new hire's performance. There's no right or wrong thing to do in the first 90 days; there's no one size fits all.

What I want my staff to do is going to be different from what you want your staff to do.

What I've just given you is a **framework** to use. It will guide you as to how you allocate your time and resources for effective training. The *Success Description* tells you what you were hiring for, and it also tells you what you're training to achieve. With your objective measures visible, you can track how well new employees are performing, and equally, how well you are coaching.

You may discover that there are a few gaps in your new hire's ability and you decide that you can train and improve them. The very worst that can happen at this point (90 days) is you realize that the person you've got is not good enough and you cut them loose.

Either way, you're in a better position than if you just let someone walk into your clinic thinking that just because they have a great resume, that they know how to solve your specific business problems. Rarely does that ever happen.

That is the last part of the ***Outcomes Based Hiring System*** completed. But we're not finished yet. Next, I want to share with you a completely AUTOMATED way of recruiting that I invented, one that has also delivered world-class staff members who I can trust.

Turn the page and read with an open mind. I think you'll be pleasantly surprised by what you're about to learn in terms of automating this process...

12

CASE STUDY: HOW TO AUTOMATE THE HIRING PROCESS

So, I've talked you through how to recruit and hire using a manual process, now let me explain how you might do it in an automated fashion.

This is a process I created a few years ago in order to limit the amount of applications I was getting in response to job ads.

I have to admit that, when I was first putting the process together, I had absolutely no idea what the results would be. But a few years on, I can tell you that it really does work. As I write this book there are three people, recruited via this process, who are currently working in my company.

What is more, I've since taught this process to hundreds of other physical therapists. This entire automated hiring system is taught in my flagship course known as *PT Business Growth School* (or BGS) – it is a 6-week online training program that shows you how to systemize and automate everything that can, and should, be automated in your business.

In this chapter, I'm giving you an overview of how the automated hiring process works. To be clear, you're still going through all of the steps I've outlined in the book. The only difference is that we're bringing the completion of tasks to the front of the interview process. As you'll soon see, the people applying through this process only make it the in-person interviews once they've followed all the steps in this mostly automated process.

TWO THINGS YOU NEED TO MAKE THIS WORK

There are two things you're going to need to have in place in order to make this work. I am introducing them to you now, even before I describe the steps, so that there's no confusion when I do.

1. CUSTOMER RELATIONSHIP MANAGEMENT SOFTWARE (CRM)

This is the automation software that runs this whole hiring campaign; without this, you cannot make it work. The one that I use, and always recommend, is Infusionsoft.

I use it for all aspects of my business, including the marketing, follow-up, sales, welcoming of patients to the clinics, and re-engaging drop offs or no-shows. It even allows me to track metrics and vital stats. If, after reading this chapter, you decide you are interested in making your clinic more automated, and you want a personal demo of how I use Infusionsoft, send an email to **paul@paulgough.com** – one of my team members will be happy to take care of you.

You can also head over to **www.paulsinfusionsoft.com** to get involved in a free training that shows you how I use it. Choose which one works best for you.

Now, once you have a CRM like Infusionsoft you can build what I call, "funnels". This is simply a marketing term for pre-written sequences of communication that patients get automatically. In the case of marketing, they enter a funnel that contains things like emails, direct mail, and even SMS text messages, all which communicate with patients about their problems (i.e. back pain).

In this case, the funnel is a sequence of communications that a prospective employee flows through. The hiring funnel is about having people interested in your job complete tasks for you in advance. They'll do so within a given time frame that proves to you that they're able to follow simple tasks.

What is more, the fact that it is mostly automated means that you can set it up once and then forget about it. When people enter the funnel they'll all receive the same emails and task, yet this happens at different times, depending on when they entered the funnel.

2. CREATE A LANDING PAGE TO COLLECT NAMES AND EMAILS

As well as Infusionsoft, the second thing that you need is something called a landing page. You need this to collect the names and contact details of the people that are interested in your job. A landing page is simply a webpage that collects data. You will have used one as a consumer when downloading things like free reports or attending webinars online. Perhaps this is how you started your relationship with me? As you request the free report, when you enter your name and email, you're on the landing page. Infusionsoft has its own landing pages and they're very easy to create.

Landing pages are commonly used in marketing when you run ads that offer people free information. To get the free information, people must first give you their contact details. When they give you the contact details, all the information gets collected by the landing page, and then it is passed on to Infusionsoft. This triggers a series of pre-written emails. It is no different here, only the content of the emails is changing.

Now, what I love about doing this is that you can use your landing page to ask for more than just a telephone number or email address. I like to ask the responding candidates some questions which let me find out more about them. For example, I might use the landing page to ask them something like this: "why are you leaving your current role", or "what are you hoping for in your new role?"

The landing page collects this and, thereafter, I am able to go into my Infusionsoft account and look at what the person has said; it becomes part of the data that I am collecting on this person, data which is helping to guide my decision. Remember, there's no one single stand-out reason that anyone should get a job with you; it is the sum of all of the data that you collect on them. The more data you collect, the better the profile you'll have about who this person really is.

Now, when the person fills out the form on the landing page, what happens next is that they'll get an instant (automated) email from me. This tells them more about the role, and most importantly, tells them what to do next. In that first email I can tell them more about the role and even include a version of the *Success Description*. I can talk about *possible* salary, *possible* working hours, my expectations, company culture, and even my vision and mission for my company. All of this is done before they go any further.

This will already separate the good from the bad and ugly. If, after reading the email they like the sound of working for you, then you ask them to do something. It could be something simple like, for example, watching a video or replying for more instructions. You can get as creative as you want and depending on the number of responses you think you're going to get, you can make it taxing or easy - controlling whether more or fewer people make it through the hoops.

And that is what we're really doing here: we're putting in a few hoops that candidates have to jump through to get to your job. How badly do they really want the job? If you've got over 100 people applying for a job (as is often the case with an admin or marketing assistant type role), then this begins to weed them out very quickly.

When I invented this "Automated Hiring Process", it was at a time when I was growing so fast that I was looking for a way to save time yet not neglect the requirements of the process. I had my physical therapy business growing strong and my worldwide marketing company was employing new people all the time, so I knew I'd be doing it again and again.

For clarity, I would not use this funnel if I had a limited number of applicants for a position. For a physical therapist, it would be a lot harder to get, say, 100 people applying for a job at any one time. What is more likely is that you'll get 5-10, and so I do not recommend that you have those applicants do automated tasks.

Understand that this process I am about to teach you should be viewed as an option; use it wisely depending upon the situation you're in and how likely it is you will be swamped with applicants.

Key point: the automated hiring system will not instantly find the right candidate; it puts you in a position to spend more time with the top five or six, so that you can choose the right one. You are still going to *create your hiring plan*, *establish the financial metric of success*, fill in the *Success Description*, and *place your ads* in as many different places as possible.

It's from this point that you're adapting the process. You are automating it, but you're still focused on **outcomes** achieved by values and skills (and not experience and personality).

With that overview complete, and now that you briefly understand how it works as well as what you'll need, let me describe exactly how I did it.

CASE STUDY: HOW I AUTOMATED THE HIRING OF A FRONT DESK PERSON FOR MY CLINIC (USING INFUSIONSOFT)

You're about to read the exact 4-step process that I used to hire a front of house/admin person for my clinic. The person whom I hired using this system is still with me as I write this book, and I am happy to report she is doing a great job. Let's get going with the steps.

STEP 1: CREATE THE LANDING PAGE

We created a landing page that looked like this:

FIG.13

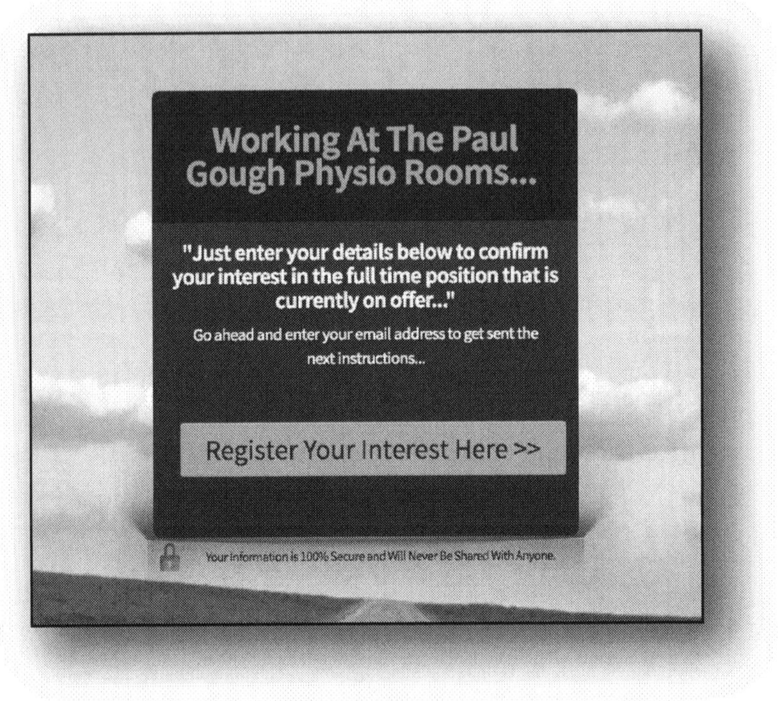
Working At The Paul Gough Physio Rooms...
"Just enter your details below to confirm your interest in the full time position that is currently on offer..."
Go ahead and enter your email address to get sent the next instructions...
Register Your Interest Here >>
Your Information is 100% Secure and Will Never Be Shared With Anyone.

Once the applicants clicked the yellow button to register interest, they were taken to the next page to enter their details. Turn the page to see how and what we ask applicants to enter…

FIG. 14 - PART 2 OF THE LANDING PAGE TO COLLECT DETAILS

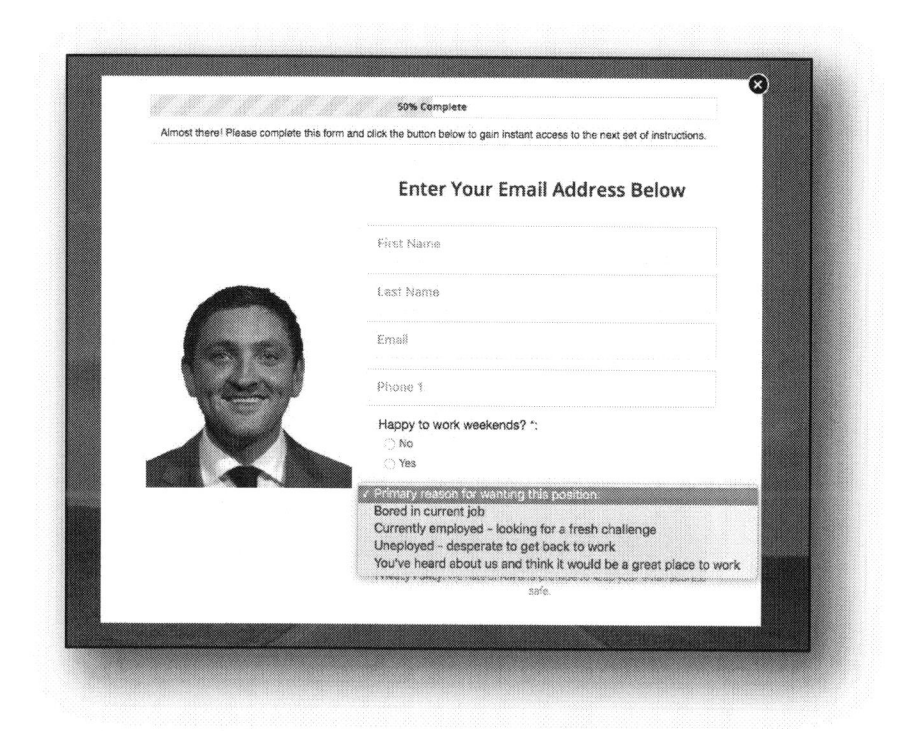

Notice what we ask for: their name and email, and, of course, telephone number. But, look what else I am asking them: "are you happy to work weekends?" Why did I ask that?

Because the job requires that they work weekends!

If they can't work weekends, or don't want to, then they won't fill out the rest of the form and that saves me more time further down the line.

What's more, I am also asking what their "primary reason for wanting this job" is, and I give them four different options to choose from. Are they bored in their current job? Looking for a fresh challenge? Have they heard about us from a patient? Their answers to the question starts to reveal something about them.

STEP 2: DISTRIBUTE TO DIFFERENT PLATFORMS

With the landing page created you can then begin circulating the job ads (covered in chapter 8) across different platforms (i.e. as many of the 11 different places covered in chapter 9).

The first platform we used was email. We started by sending an email to our patient database with the subject line, "we're hiring." This was a 500-word email announcing to thousands of people on my clinic database that there was a position vacant at my clinic. It gave a brief overview of the job and told them what to do if they were interested; simply fill out the form and wait for the next steps by email.

We created ads for use on social media whilst circulating them across all of our clinic's networks. And, we also asked all of the staff to share them out. Here's what the ad looked like:

FIG.15

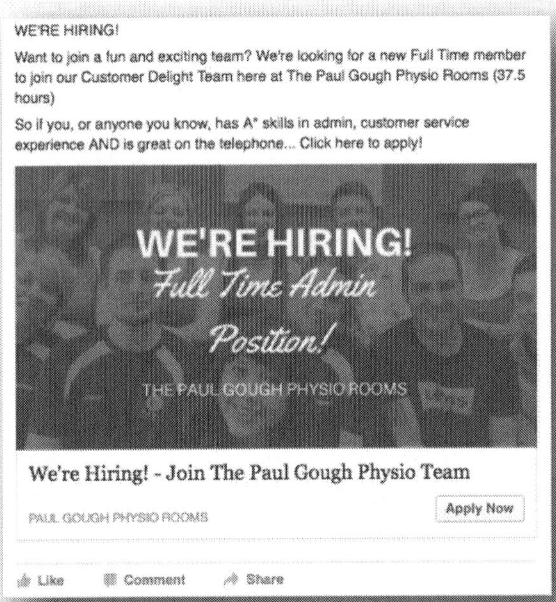

WE'RE HIRING!

Want to join a fun and exciting team? We're looking for a new Full Time member to join our Customer Delight Team here at The Paul Gough Physio Rooms (37.5 hours)

So if you, or anyone you know, has A* skills in admin, customer service experience AND is great on the telephone... Click here to apply!

WE'RE HIRING!
Full Time Admin Position!
THE PAUL GOUGH PHYSIO ROOMS

We're Hiring! - Join The Paul Gough Physio Team

PAUL GOUGH PHYSIO ROOMS — Apply Now

Like   Comment   Share

Again, all that applicants had to do was click the ad, taking them to the landing page, and from there they could leave us their details.

STEP 3: SEND THE INSTRUCTIONS USING EMAIL

Once the candidates filled out the form and gave us their details, they were immediately sent an email. The first email that they got requested that they watch a video.

In this case study, I had them watch a video of my staff answering the common FAQ's of physical therapy. It is the same video that we send to patients when they first book appointments with us. Here's where this gets interesting: the candidate only made it to the next part of the process if they clicked and watched the video.

The great thing about Infusionsoft is that it allows you to see how people interact with your email; you can use something called "tags", which get applied if people open emails or click to watch videos. I can even find out how long they watched the video for.

Assuming that they watched the video, the automation continued and the next email went out at 12pm the following day. For those who didn't watch the video in the first step, they didn't get anything else from me. They were removed from the rest of the funnel.

WEED OUT THE TIME WASTERS

Here's the power of doing this: in this real life case study, the initial applicant pool was 147. That number dropped to 37 within the first 24 hours. This is because, of the 147 who said they were interested – having filled out the landing page from the email or social media post – 110 didn't follow the instructions in the email; they didn't even click to watch the video.

Here's why this is important:

If I'd interviewed all of those 110 people and asked them how willing and keen they were to work for me, they'd all have said "very". If I'd have asked each one of the 110, "would you be willing to learn, watch videos in your own time, and go over and above for my business?", they'd have all said "yes".

There's a big difference between <u>what people say</u> and <u>what people do,</u> and this process highlights it perfectly.

So, what happened next was the group of 37 (who clicked to watch the video in the first email) were all sent another email containing another set of instructions. This happened the next day at 12pm.

In this email I asked them all to write a **575-600 word** letter that would/could be sent to a prospective patient. This letter was meant to answer one or two questions that were covered in the video they watched the day before. I wanted them to write a letter explaining why Paul Gough Physio Rooms would be a great place to go for physical therapy and the letter had to be sent back to us <u>within 24 hours.</u>

These tasks are asking applicants to show me <u>proof</u> of their abilities, that is, proof that they will do the things required in the job.

If someone got the role, they would have to answer questions from patients about physical therapy; the applicant is going to have to be able to "sell" the value of my clinic from that front desk role. Why not ask the candidates to demonstrate how well they can do it before you give them the job?

As well as answer common FAQ's, they're also going to have to write letters to patients and doctors, and this task is going to give me proof of how good (or bad) their writing skills are. Are there any spelling or grammatical errors?

But mostly, what this task does is provide me with a 'check box' of sorts, to see if they can follow basic instructions. Can they get the letter back within 24 hours? Did they send it to the right email address? Or, did they just reply to the one that was used to send them their instructions?

By the way, many did send it to the wrong email. Many actually sent back a letter with 2000 words while some wrote even less than 300. In the task they were asked for 575-600 words for a reason. That's because I wanted a letter with between 575 and 600 words in it. Again, I was testing to see how well they could follow instructions.

All of these are giving me clues as to who this person really is; I am learning how attentive they really are; how committed they really are. I am not basing my judgment solely off of who they say they are.

This second task narrowed down the pool of candidates to just 14. This is where it got really fun: the next thing we did was to ask all of those 14 candidates to record a video talking about themselves for 7 minutes. Why did I do this? It's because the role they were applying for was in my front of house (admin) team. I believe the most important part of that role is not how efficient the person is with paper work, sending emails or answering the phone, but how well they can talk to my patients and put them at ease when they walk through the doors.

That is their job!

If they do that well, then they solve a lot of my problems. What is more, I've studied my patients for years; I've been analyzing their moves and studying their questions and behavior patterns when they walk through my doors. One of the most striking observations is how long it can take some people to feel comfortable in a new environment.

Some are at ease right away, but for others it can take a little while to get comfortable enough to even go beyond a "yes" or "no" type conversation. I worked out that, for many people coming into the clinic, it could take them about 5-7 minutes before feeling comfortable enough to talk openly and freely.

If you want a quick example of what I mean, try asking your patients if they want a cup of coffee or tea. To the ones who say "no thank you", ask them again... and then again... usually, at about around the third time, the ones who said "no" will say "oh, go on then".

Why did that happen? They didn't all of a sudden just get thirsty or need a caffeine hit in the last five seconds. It was because when they first answered, they didn't feel comfortable. That is how most people start relationships with most companies. That's not how I want it in my company, though. That's why it is the job of the front of house person to be able to recognize when someone is uncomfortable – and change it. If they don't, you've got a very cold and uncomfortable patient sitting in silence in a waiting room.

That is not a good position to be in when the patient is soon to make a decision about their health and spending money with you. Anyone who understands the psychology of selling, (and buying), knows that this is the worst situation for a buyer to be in.

People who are cold, and who feel uncomfortable, do not make good decisions. Patients who feel this way make rash, often irrational decisions and do not proceed with treatment. And their preferred excuse? Cost.

The real reason is not cost though, it's that they are not comfortable enough to spend money with you. You don't change this in the treatment room, you change it *before* they enter the treatment room. It's why I say that it's in the reception area that the real money is made.

Sure, the physical therapists have the clinical skills, but it is the front desk person who can, and should, be putting the patient at ease so that the physical therapists job is made easier. People do not buy from a place of logic (i.e. clinical skills), they buy from a place of emotion. For example, people do don't buy new shoes because they need them. No, they buy them because they look better with the new jeans they've just bought than the old ones do.

That's why you must find or have someone in your clinic who has this ability to be comfortable with talking to people who, at first, might be uncomfortable and do not want to talk back. It takes a certain type of person to not take offense or feel insecure when someone doesn't appear to want to talk or engage with them at first. I am looking for precisely that person. That's why I asked people to record a video and send it back to me; to show me that they're happy to step outside of their comfort zone.

Asking people to record a 7-minute video showed me whether the person applying was comfortable talking for this period of time. Do they have that skill? And, as a happy by-product, it also showed me if the applicants could figure something out that they might not know how to do like, for example, record and send in a video.

Many people would never have done something like this before. They'll have been forced to seek help or advice from a friend or a family member, and this told me something else about them: are they willing to go over and above to get the task done?

ALWAYS TELL THEM WHY YOU NEED THEM TO DO IT

Of course, in all of the emails I explained why we needed them to do these things. We linked it all back to the core values of the business and explained that we are very clear on what we are about and because of that we have a certain type of person in mind for the role.

We told the candidates that anyone who recorded this video and sent it to us on time would automatically be guaranteed an interview. Now I was left with just five candidates.

With these five candidates lined up, I was able to pick up the hiring process from the *in-person interview* phase (that I described in chapter 10). Each one of these five candidates was invited for their first in-person interview. From that I was able to narrow the list down further to three people, all of whom I invited back for interview number two.

From that group, I then selected the strongest candidate, and, finally, I arrived at a candidate who has since been with me for over two years. That person is a valuable member of my team who I would never want to lose.

Bottom line… the process works. As well as front desk people, I've since used it to hire marketing assistants in my marketing company. The only thing that changes about the process is the specific task I am asking them to do which is obviously more specific to marketing.

In the case of a marketing assistant, I asked them to send a social media marketing campaign for my clinic, record and edit a video, and explain how they would use Facebook or Google Ads to find patients for my clinic. These are all of the tasks they would be required to do if/when an applicant got the job.

It's like I keep stressing, if you're clear about what it is that you want people to do for you, hiring is easy; you can get very creative with this process, and what is more, the right candidates are excited by it.

I received a couple of emails from people who didn't like the fact that I was asking them to do these tasks, and simultaneously, I received just as many emails saying how different it was, how they'd never seen anything like it before, and how they loved it. They were excited at the prospect of working for such a forward thinking and progressive company. Remember when I said one of the rules of hiring was to "repel and attract"? Well, this process does that as well.

WANT TO GET THIS ENTIRE HIRING FUNNEL?

If you like the sound of this process, this has just been an overview. The entire *Automated Hiring System* is broken down in my **PT Business Growth School 6-week online training program**. You get all of the emails, ads, videos, instructions, and processes that I used to make this work and which 100's of other clinic owners have also made work for them.

When you enroll in the class you'll get to work with me personally and you'll also get help setting it all up, not to mention you'll be receiving an additional five other modules all dedicated to systems and automating your clinic. Check out the *PT Business Growth School* program here: **www.paulsbgs.com**

What's more, if you're interested in using Infusionsoft to automate and systemize your clinic, my team can recreate this entire funnel bespoke for you and your needs. For free training on how I use Infusionsoft, go to: **www.paulsinfusionsoft.com.** Alternately, request a personal demo consultation by emailing **paul@paulgough.com.**

We can have this automated hiring funnel along with marketing, sales, past patient re-activation, and other funnels at your fingertips inside 30 days from now.

13

• •

YOUR OPPORTUNITY TO WORK WITH PAUL BEYOND THIS BOOK

So, there you have it: precisely how to recruit, hire, and train world-class people whom you can trust to grow your clinic.

If you're looking to hire, then it's obvious that you're growing or want to grow. The question is, **do you want to grow with ease and maximum profitability?** If you do, then I'd like to offer you my help.

Anyone who picks up a book on hiring is obviously looking to bring in more people. And, the goal of doing that is surely to allow you to grow a more successful clinic? Well, to do that, the next thing that you need to is to create the systems for your business that these new hires can run for you.

Ultimately, people do not run businesses, <u>systems do</u>. And it is your job as the owner of the business to create those systems.

To grow a successful business you need **leverage;** you will get that from your marketing message, from hiring the right people, and having automated systems which allow you, as the owner of the business, to spend more time doing high value/high dollar work.

I can help you with all of that. And there are two ways that we can work together beyond this book:

OPTION 1 – FREE ONLINE TRAINING

"Automating Growth: How to Automate and Systemize Everything in Your Clinic for Explosive Growth and Profits"

This webinar is free for you to attend; it's an in-depth online training that gives you a behind-the-scenes look at the systems I've used to scale my clinic from one premises, to four. I also show you how I automate everything that can possibly be automated, meaning I have a more profitable, easily run business – one which grows without me.

The 90-minute webinar will show you the types of systems you'll need if you want to grow and scale with ease. My clinic moved away from the "manual" stuff a long time ago that leaves most clinic owners tired and burned out – and we've never looked back.

If you want a fully automated and systemized clinic, this webinar is a great place for you to start. I will be hosting the free online training personally, and you will be able to submit your questions to me beforehand.

HERE'S WHAT YOU'LL LEARN WHEN YOU ATTEND:

- Precisely how to leverage "automation" so that your PT business grows without you.

- The top 5 most important "Clinic Growth Systems" and how to use them to grow your practice profits

- How to find more time for spending with family AND patients

- The 7 secret "automation" aspects of my business that have helped me grow and scale with ease (no matter what country I'm in).

- "Marketing Automation" – it's NEW, it's effortless, and I'll show you "2" ways to put it to work in your business; with this, you'll pick up new patients 24/7.

- Success Stories: how other clinic owners have copied my system for explosive clinic growth… and you can do the same!

TAKE THE FREE TRAINING HERE:

WWW.PAULSAUTOMATIONWEBINAR.COM

OPTION 2 – FREE ONLINE TRAINING

WORK WITH ME IN MY PHYSICAL THERAPY BUSINESS GROWTH SCHOOL PROGRAM

Physical Therapy Business Growth School is the advanced 6-week systems and automation training that I designed to help businesses grow and scale faster.

It gives you everything that you need to create a fully automated and systemized clinic – one that grows and runs without you. I go much deeper on the free training, and I give you all of the templates, scripts, emails, hiring ads, and spreadsheets that you'll need to do it.

This is not theory – it is fact! If you know my story well, you'll know that I am rarely in my own clinic, yet it continues to run without me. The fact that my clinic continues to create a six-figure profit even though I am rarely in the country these days is not so much to do with me, but everything to do with the **systems** I created.

As I said earlier, people do not run businesses – systems do. And it is the people you hire that run those systems for you. The better the systems, the less hassle you'll get as you grow, and what's more, the more profitable you'll be!

Now you know how to get the right people – *PT Business Growth School* shows you how to create the right systems and how to have them run on your behalf.

Tip: do not hire people without having the right infrastructure, as they'll quickly become more of a liability than an asset. For most business owners, growth brings bigger headaches, more hassles, and a smaller profit margin. It doesn't have to be that way, and on this program I show you how I avoided that trap. I also show you how 100's of clinic owners, much like you, have been able to do the same thing I did since taking this class with me.

Most people tell me that they "want systems" in their clinic, and yet, when I ask which ones, they have no clue. Can you relate? Do you know you need systems, but are just not sure which ones, or even where to start?

In this class, I'll not only show you the key systems that will generate more profit, fix leaks, and leverage automation (saving time), but I'll give you most of the things that you're going to need to create those systems with ease.

I'll give you all of the **front desk scripts** and **evaluation scripts for PTs**, and I'll walk you through the **entire patient journey experience,** giving you **example emails, videos,** and **process maps and blueprints** to plug all of this into your business in less than 6 weeks.

I'll help you create, and then implement, the **right values in your clinic. I'll show you how to establish and communicate**

your clinic's USP – right throughout your clinic. And, there's an entire seminar on the **essential financial principles** that every clinic owner needs to know in order to run a profitable business.

What's more, I also spend an entire seminar showing you how to create the automated hiring funnel that we covered in chapter 12. We'll go deeper into how to implement the automated hiring funnel, and you'll **get the exact emails, videos, and instructions that we send to the candidates who go through the process; and all of *this* is a special bonus for signing up through this book!**

With this program you'll get high level business coaching from me – plus the physical material you'll need to create the key systems in record time.

You'll have access to me throughout the program, and this is the same program that has allowed 100's of clinic owners to **stop doing $10 per hour work** in order to focus on $500 per hour work, instead.

This program has helped solo-practitioners get to clinic owner status with new employees coming into a fully systemized clinic allowing the owner more time to work *ON* it, and not be trapped *IN* it.

It is the same program that has helped PT Carrie Jose, of Portsmouth, New Hampshire, go from solo practitioner – stuck in a tiny treatment room in a rented facility, working day and night without anyone or anything to help her – to becoming the proud owner of her own business with its own facility. She now employs staff and has record growth year-on-year since taking the class.

It is the same program that helped Jason Han, of HealthFit. in Pasadena, Ca, to go from working all day and all night in his small practice, to owning a bigger, more profitable practice which now has more staff doing the work for him. He is now free to spend more time with his baby daughter and beautiful young family.

Head over to this page, **www.paulsbgs.com** here, you'll be able to hear about their stories in full.

Best of all, this is the program that has helped 100's of clinic owners who were feeling stuck and burned out – doing the same thing day after day with little, if any, additional profit no matter how hard they worked – to escape that dreadful way of living they call the "Rat Race".

It's a 6-week program dedicated to showing you how to create systems that leverage automation, meaning you can grow a business with ease. And if you wanted, you wouldn't even have to be there every day.

Whether you are a brand new start-up or an established business stuck and wanting to grow, this program is perfect for you, and there's never a better time than NOW to **automate and put the right systems into your clinic.**

HERE'S WHAT WE'LL COVER TOGETHER IN THE PROGRAM:

- How to auto-pilot and systemize EVERYTHING in your business so that it grows without you. This is critical to your business growth. We'll cover how to onboard new patients, evaluation scripts, stopping drop-offs and re-activating past patients, getting a "yes" – even if they say "no" – and getting referrals within 72 hours!

- Marketing Automation – it's now the easiest and fastest way to grow a PT clinic (...PLUS, it's a lot less time-consuming and costly than marketing to local doctors).

- How to spend more time with family – and still make the same money

- How to build a world-class team that runs your business for you (using the systems you'll be creating...).

- How to break-free of your business's "daily grind" and transfer important responsibilities to others – getting "you" out of your own way!

- How to find, hire, and train a complete replacement for yourself so you can step aside from being a PT….to leading a team!

- How to grow and manage from multiple sites (and the technology you can leverage to make it easier).

- How to move beyond systems that are outdated, maxed out, or ones that you've simply outgrown (so that your growth is not being limited technologically).

- How to make the jump from solo-PT to having a team (...and how to know when it's time to make the change).

How to maintain your business's culture, personality, and clinical EXCELLENCE as you grow (and how to know if/when a brand change is needed).

Everything you need is delivered to you via a series of instant access videos, PDF scripts, live Q/A calls (with me), and an interactive online community (of hundreds of other *PT Business Growth School* students); all of *this* is to ensure that you can install these systems – which leverage automation – into your clinic without any hassle or getting stuck.

ACCESS THE ADVANCED SYSTEMS AND AUTOMATION MASTERCLASS, HERE:

WWW.PAULSBGS.COM

This is an instant training – you can start TODAY. And, if after reading this book you have decided that you not only want to hire the best people who you can trust, **but that you want the right SYSTEMS that anyone can run**, then this is perfect for you.

Do not wait another minute to get these systems into your business – go ahead and start the class now. Do that here:

WWW.PAULSBGS.COM

To your success,

Paul Gough

P.S Here's what people have to say about this remarkable *Physical Therapy Business Growth School* program, now known to many around the world as "BGS":

"I don't know where I would be without The Physical Therapy Business Growth School. In the space of 2 years we have grown from a team of two, to seven, our income has more than double in less than a year, and we're working less!"
Jason Han, HealthFit, Los Angeles, CA

"At the time of taking Business Growth School, I had no plans to open up my own space, mostly because I didn't believe I could! Since implementing what Paul has taught me in growth school about hiring and systems, I've moved into my own space. My monthly revenue has tripled, it's never dropped, and is continuing to grow! I have a strong team I can trust and an amazing community of clients who are a joy to work with and truly enjoy coming to see us."
Carrie Jose, CJ Physical Therapy and Pilates, Portsmouth, NH

You can hear these phenomenal business owners speak in their own words about how this program has impacted them. Just go to this page:

WWW.PAULSBGS.COM

ABOUT THE AUTHOR

PAUL GOUGH is the No.1 bestselling author of *The New Patient Accelerator Method*, a revolutionary new marketing book for physical therapists; he's also an international speaker and a former professional soccer physical therapist turned successful clinic owner from the UK. Paul is the founder of the *Paul Gough Physio Rooms* – a successful **four location cash pay clinic** that he started from a spare room in his home whilst having had no money and no business or marketing skills. Paul has since scaled his clinic from a zero to $1m +, and what's most impressive is that he's done all that in a country with a completely free, "socialist" health care system (one that provides physical therapy services for FREE for all UK residents) as his main competitor.

He is a true small business success story; he is now the owner of five companies, all of which are in three different markets and in two different countries – two of those companies have achieved million dollar+ revenues.

Paul is the host of the top-rated podcast *The Physical Therapy Business School Podcast* (available on iTunes, Soundcloud and Stitcher). He is also a "Small Business ICON" WINNER of the *Infusionsoft* award for best in 'class lead nurture marketing' in 2016, an award which is selected from all across Infusionsoft's 45,000+ global customers.

He is widely regarded, both in America and around the world, as a leading authority on direct to consumer marketing, and he has a proven track record of helping physical therapists attract cash pay patients, growing their practices, increasing profits, freeing up their time, and radically shifting their entrepreneurial thinking. Every week, 10,000's of physical therapists receive his support/advice online and attend his seminars. His business success coaching programs are almost always full.

BE SURE TO CONNECT WITH PAUL ON SOCIAL MEDIA AND LET HIM KNOW HOW THIS BOOK MADE AN IMPACT ON YOU: @THEPAULGOUGH

OTHER BOOKS BY PAUL GOUGH

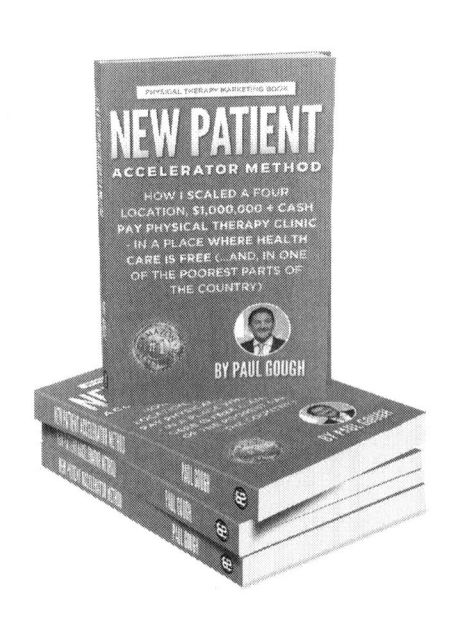

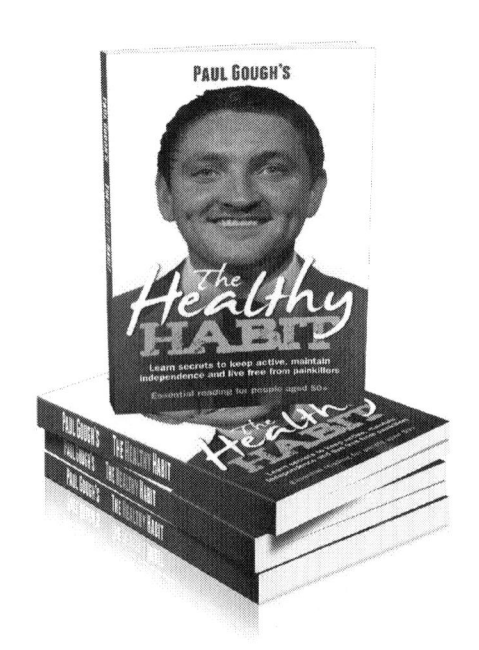

New Patient Accelerator Method:
www.paulsmarketingbook.com

The Healthy Habit:
www.thehealthyhabitbook.com

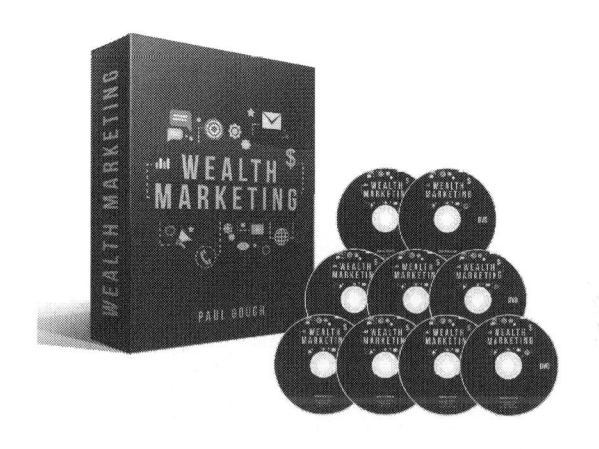

GET YOUR FREE WEALTH MARKETING GIFT FROM PAUL, NOW...

Go to: **www.paulgough.com/wealth-gift**
To get this instant access 9 DVD video program, NOW

Claim your $1,997.00 worth of cash patient generating, higher profit making, wealth marketing DVD program, absolutely FREE!

Including a FREE "Test-Drive" of Paul Gough's Cash Club Membership that sends to your clinic $10,000 worth of marketing ideas every 30 days.

**Claim your copy now, at
www.paulgough.com/wealth-gift**

Printed in Great Britain
by Amazon